NURSING HISTORY REVIEW

OFFICIAL JOURNAL OF THE AMERICAN ASSOCIATION FOR THE
HISTORY OF NURSING   1996 · Volume 4
University of Pennsylvania Press   ISSN 1062-8061

CONTENTS

DOING THE WORK OF HISTORY

BOOK REVIEWS

Volume 4   1996

Nursing History Review

Copyright © 1996 by The American Association for the History of Nursing

Nursing History Review is published annually for the American Association for the History of Nursing, Inc., by the University of Pennsylvania Press.

International Standard Serial Number ISSN 1062-8061
International Standard Book Number ISBN 0-8122-1453-6 (Volume 4)
Printed in the United States of America

All inquiries concerning subscriptions or advertising should be sent to:

Marketing Department
University of Pennsylvania Press
423 Guardian Drive
Philadelphia, Pa. 19104-6097
Attention: Subscription Manager

Yearly subscription rates are: $36.00, individuals; $55.00, institutions and libraries.

Members of the American Association for the History of Nursing, Inc. (AAHN) receive *Nursing History Review* on payment of $60.00 annual membership dues. Applications and other correspondence relating to AAHN membership should be directed to:

Dr. Rosemary McCarthy, Executive Director
American Association for the History of Nursing, Inc.
P.O. Box 90803
Washington, D.C. 20090-0803

Please direct all submissions and editorial correspondence to:

Joan E. Lynaugh, Editor
Nursing History Review
University of Pennsylvania
420 Guardian Drive, Room 307
Philadelphia, Pa. 19104-6096

Articles appearing in *Nursing History Review* are indexed in *Cumulative Index to Nursing & Allied Health Literature*, *Current Contents/Social & Behavioral Sciences*, *Social Sciences Citation Index*, *Research Alert*, *RNdex*, and in *Index Medicus* and MEDLINE on the National Library of Medicine's MEDLARS system. They are also abstracted and indexed in *Historical Abstracts* and *America: History and Life*.

Printed on acid-free paper, effective with Volume 1 (1993).

Cover photo: Linda Richards in Japan. The Japanese woman accompanying Richards may have been a graduate of the first class who became Richards's assistant and her first teacher of Japanese. (From the Linda Richards Collection, Boston University Libraries. By permission of Nursing Archives, Mugar Memorial Library.)

NURSING HISTORY REVIEW

JOAN E. LYNAUGH, Editor
BARBARA BRODIE, Book Review Editor
WENDY WASHBURN, Assistant Editor

Editorial Review Board

Ellen D. Baer
New York

Susan Baird
Fox Chase Cancer Center
Pennsylvania

Nettie Birnbach
Florida

Barbara Brodie
University of Virginia
Virginia

Olga Maranjian Church
University of Connecticut
Connecticut

Donna Diers
Yale University
Connecticut

Marilyn Flood
University of California
at San Francisco
California

Diane Hamilton
Western Michigan State
Michigan

Beatrice Kalisch
University of Michigan
Michigan

Eloise Lewis
North Carolina

Mary Ann Lewis
University of California
at Los Angeles
California

Susan Reverby
Wellesley College
Massachusetts

Nancy Tomes
SUNY at Stony Brook
New York

EDITORIAL

You will find carefully researched historical narratives in this volume of *Nursing History Review* which span time from 1800 to our own generation and traverse the globe from Canada to China. The word for nursing and its history is "ubiquitous." So, why do we still meet colleagues who insist that studying history is a waste of time? "History," they say, "is rather nice to know, adds a bit of polish and interest, but it is so impractical." Then they ask, "How do you expect to get ahead, to get your research funded, to get a job?" What follows is my brief defense of our subject.

History is our source of identity, our cultural DNA; it affords us collective immortality. History yields self-knowledge by structuring a mind capable of imagining life beyond one's own life-span. History continuously proposes new ideas, values, and experiences, thus creating and recreating culture and discipline. History explains connections and patterns among events. The chronology of history enables historians to interpret events inside contextual frames; we, in turn, are able to grasp meaning, achieve perspective, and avoid ill-informed or random judgment.

History fills our minds, so we enjoy it for its own sake; it helps us gain identity and personal meaning in our work, improves our comprehension and our planning, and validates social criticism. History makes better sense of the present and helps us project a more coherent vision of the future. As historian Arthur Schlesinger put it, "History supplies the antidote to every generation's illusion that its own problems are uniquely oppressive."

Or, you can just show them Volume 4.

JOAN E. LYNAUGH

Center for the Study of the History of Nursing
University of Pennsylvania

ARTICLES

Backrubs vs. Bach
Nursing and the Entry-into-Practice Debate, 1946–1986

SUSAN RIMBY LEIGHOW
History Department
Shippensburg University

In 1966 Patricia Early wrote an indignant letter to the *American Journal of Nursing* (*AJN*), protesting a recent Position Paper on Education issued by the American Nurses Association (ANA). Nurse Early, a graduate of a hospital training school, expressed hostility toward a statement made by the ANA. A year earlier the ANA had recommended that all future registered nurses (RNs) be educated in colleges and universities. Nurse Early, concerned with the proposal's impact on both RNs and patients, issued a challenge to the ANA's leaders. "Please prove to me that I can give a better back rub or enema by taking courses in music appreciation or literature."[1]

Patricia Early's letter was only one salvo in a battle that nurses had fought almost since the inception of the profession. Since the 1890s, the leadership and the rank and file differed over the issue of entry-level training. Several historians have documented the class-based nature of the debate, which pitted upper- and middle-class leaders in education, administration, and public health against working-class private duty nurses and hospital staff. Leaders' calls for higher educational standards masked a concern about the rank and file's roots and the occupation's servile status. Professional associations' attempts to upgrade hospital schools and later to establish collegiate programs were designed to restrict the numbers of RNs, recruit women of higher social standing, and ultimately raise wages and prestige. Rank-and-file nurses vigorously fought these changes.[2]

Nursing History Review 4 (1996): 3–17. Copyright © 1996 by The American Association for the History of Nursing.

As historians have also shown, this debate was largely moot. The leadership possessed few allies and they lacked a rationale for educational reform. American society saw nursing as a logical extension of women's work, not as a scientific profession.[3]

After World War II

After 1945, however, the entry-into-practice issue took on new life. Postwar trends in both nursing and the larger American society made educational reform feasible. The nature of the debate also changed. Although discussion on attracting better qualified women did not completely disappear, it became less elitist. Nursing leaders also used other arguments.

The rank and file, however, remained skeptical about entry-level college education. They defended traditional practices and were suspicious of their leaders' motives. A large number of nurses fought educational reform well into the 1980s.[4] The entry-into-practice issue continued to divide nursing, even as the circumstances that had originally triggered the controversy changed. The often bitter debate, waged at ANA conventions and in the pages of the professional press, proved that postwar leaders and rank-and-file RNs still held widely divergent opinions.

Like the majority of prewar Americans, nurses in the United States largely bypassed college. As late as 1945, 99 percent of RNs received their initial professional education in hospital schools.[5] These programs, first established in the United States during the early 1870s, provided students with an apprenticeship. Under this system, young women lived within the hospital for a period ranging from six months to three years and learned how to nurse by practicing required skills on the institution's patients.

Critics charged that hospitals used these women as a source of cheap labor, provided little in the way of formal education, and graduated students ill-prepared to practice.[6] Early-twentieth-century nursing leaders, conscious of the oversupply of practitioners, also blamed small schools with short training programs for accepting unqualified applicants and flooding the market.[7] The leadership had little success in solving these dilemmas.

Educational Reform

Post–World War II circumstances made educational reform more compelling. Demographic trends such as longer life expectancy and the baby boom

changed the health needs of the U.S. population.[8] This population growth dramatically increased the number of Americans who were susceptible to illness and needed preventive health services. Public health nurses who could treat school-aged children and perform home care for the elderly were needed as much as hospital staff.[9] At the same time, group medical insurance and a postwar hospital construction boom made medical treatment more accessible and affordable.[10]

Advances in areas such as pharmacology, psychiatry, and cardiac care expanded the number of people in medical treatment and multiplied the number of procedures performed on patients.[11] They also dramatically altered nursing practice. Postwar RNs administered innovative drug therapies, used new intensive-care techniques, and nursed complicated surgical cases. Physicians increasingly delegated complex procedures such as closed-chest heart massage.[12] These situations presented nurses with new responsibilities and required independent decision-making. In the words of historian Barbara Melosh, "No critical care nurse would call a doctor to report meekly, 'Mr. Brown's pulse appears to have ceased.' She would yell for emergency equipment, pound the patient's chest, inflate his lungs, initiate closed-chest massage, perhaps even begin to administer the drugs used in resuscitation."[13] At the same time, increased use of practical nurses and aides to perform hospitals' housekeeping chores required RNs to become supervisors and to develop administrative and managerial skills.[14]

While nursing faced these challenges, American higher education also underwent tremendous change. Pre–World War II universities had served a primarily upper-middle-class clientele.[15] After 1945, Cold War–inspired fear spurred the recruitment of the brightest students, leading to increased federal and state aid to colleges. Educational institutions expanded enrollments, broadened curricula, and removed many barriers to matriculation. The G.I. Bill, the civil rights movement, and the establishment of community colleges further aided the expansion of higher education. Universal college attendance became a desirable social goal.[16] By the 1970s, 50 percent of American youth attended institutions of higher learning.[17]

Scientific Basis for Practice

Nursing leaders were aware of these developments and used them to advance the case for educational reform. Before World War II, proponents "did not argue that educational reform would enhance nurses' scientific understanding of health and disease."[18] After the war, the leadership stated

TABLE 1.   PERCENTAGE OF STUDENTS ENROLLED IN ENTRY-LEVEL NURSING
EDUCATION PROGRAMS, 1945–1985.

	Diploma[a]	ADN[b]	BSN[c]
1945	95	NA[d]	5
1950	93	NA	7
1955	85	2	13
1960	79	3	18
1965	65	11	24
1970	38	30	32
1975	24	36	40
1980	17	41	42
1985	14	44	42

Sources: Data from ANA, Facts About Nursing, 1951 (New York: ANA, 1951), 41; ANA, Facts About Nursing, 1957 (New York: ANA, 1957), 67; ANA, Facts About Nursing, '76–'77 (Kansas City: ANA, 1977), 97; ANA, Facts About Nursing, '80–'81 (New York: AJN Company, 1981), 152; and ANA, Facts About Nursing, 86–87 (New York: ANA, 1987), 38.
[a] Diploma graduates are nurses who completed a hospital nursing school's course of training.
[b] Nurses with an associate degree (ADN) graduated from a two-year community or junior college.
[c] Nurses with a baccalaureate degree (BSN) graduated from a four-year college or university.
[d] ADN programs were not widely available until the mid-1950s.

that complex health care technology required a new type of RN who could be educated only in the university. They also argued that nursing needed to reform educational programs in order to recruit the increasing numbers of college-bound American youth. The Russell Sage Foundation's 1947 report on nursing education buttressed these rationales, and a serious postwar RN shortage made the arguments more compelling.[19]

In the late 1940s, the major American nursing associations began campaigning extensively for educational reform. Both the ANA and the National League for Nursing (NLN) lobbied successfully for public funds. During the late 1940s and 1950s, federal and state governments passed legislation designed to aid nursing graduate students. Beginning with the passage of the landmark Nurse Training Act in 1964, Congress funded the establishment of colleges and undergraduate nursing education.[20] Literally thousands of American nursing students benefited from the expansion of college programs and government-financed scholarships, grants, and loans. Roughly 77 percent of postwar undergraduates and 40 percent of nursing graduate students could not have attended school without such aid.[21]

In some parts of the country, particularly in California, nursing leaders

in the 1950s also supported the development of community college associate degree programs. They reasoned that community college students, freed from the hospital schools' heavy workloads, learned nursing in an educationally sound environment. Because community colleges charged low tuition and graduated RNs in two years, they were also financially feasible for students unable to afford a university program or unwilling to spend four years in school.[22]

As a result of these trends, aspiring students found college more accessible than ever before. Between 1945 and 1985 the number of four-year undergraduate nursing programs more than tripled and community college schools increased almost eightfold. Nursing provided upward mobility for women as the number of women enrolled in entry-level collegiate nursing schools expanded rapidly. By 1970, 62 percent of nursing students attended associate degree and baccalaureate programs. By 1985 that figure had risen to 86 percent (see Table 1).

College Education

The professional associations attempted to codify these trends. In May 1965, one year after the passage of the Nurse Training Act, NLN delegates passed Resolution 5, which "recognized and strongly supported the trend toward collegiate nursing."[23] In December of that same year, the ANA Board of Directors issued its Position Paper on Education which endorsed the following proposals:

> The education for all those who are licensed to practice nursing should take place in institutions of higher education. Minimum preparation for beginning professional nursing practice at the present time should be baccalaureate degree education in nursing. Minimum preparation for beginning technical [bedside] nursing practice at the present time should be associate degree education in nursing.[24]

During the late 1960s, the 1970s, and the early 1980s, the associations attempted to implement their proposals. They called for the closure of hospital schools, sought accreditation changes, and lobbied state governments for a two-track licensure system.[25] The pronouncements of nursing leaders and the growth of collegiate nursing touched off a wave of protest from rank-and-file nurses. Angry hospital graduates fought attempts to mandate college degrees and pressured the ANA and NLN to rescind

their positions.[26] By the 1980s, community college graduates, upset about the proposed two-track licensure system, also voiced concern about the leadership's intentions. While associate degree nurses supported educational reform, they also feared being relegated to second-class status.[27] The associations failed to meet the ANA's proposed goal of mandating college education by 1985.[28] The debate over educational reform scarred the professional associations and left an atmosphere of hostility in its wake.

Entry-into-Practice Debate Escalates

Why, despite the changes in nursing and the growing accessibility of college education, did this entry-into-practice debate continue to create dissension? The problem persisted because nursing leaders and the rank and file continued to hold very different beliefs about the nature and purpose of professional training. The leaders, joined now by the growing number of university-educated nurses, stated the case in terms of the need for scientific education. Associate degree graduates, while ambivalent about proposed licensure changes, also made statements about the superiority of college education. In addition, nursing leaders used a modified "better class of women" argument. They pointed to the growing number of college students and argued that qualified applicants were not interested in apprenticeship training. Raising educational standards, they argued, was also the best way to make working conditions attractive to modern American women.

The rank and file, however, talked in terms of traditional nursing skills and service to the patient. Hospital graduates believed the new trends demeaned the bedside nurse's expertise and replaced dedication and experience with an unnecessary and dangerous emphasis on credentials. These women, like those earlier in the century, were suspicious of their leaders' intentions and feared that reform threatened their own status.

Real-World Clinical Experiences vs. Academia

Supporters of apprenticeship education who wrote in the nursing journals between 1946 and 1986 emphasized the importance of craft skills and quality patient care. Training-school graduates proudly defended the virtues of hospital-based education. These included the opportunity to practice tech-

niques and tricky manual procedures until they became second nature, and the chance to work on the wards and benefit from the advice of seasoned veterans.[29] They wholeheartedly agreed with the nurse who wrote in 1966 that "nursing in the true sense of the word is an art that can be perfected with some education, good supervision, and a lot of practice."[30] For women schooled in the apprenticeship system, hospital-based education instilled confidence, good judgment, and something college education could never duplicate — "adequate practical experience, something you don't get out of books or classrooms."[31]

Nurses from the hospital programs cited the advantages of their schools from another angle — the wide variety of real-world experiences they offered. They argued that college students, sheltered in the halls of academia, did not receive such experience. One hospital graduate and staff nurse, writing to the *AJN* in 1967, lambasted the colleges for their failure to incorporate shift rotation into student clinical practice. She wondered, "How can nurses possibly get the total picture of patient care when as students they work only in the mornings? Patients often feel worse in the evening and during the night."[32] Other nurses stated that the hospital courses provided more breadth and depth in nursing, while college programs included too many irrelevant subjects at the expense of nursing arts. One woman who was upset with the ANA Position Paper mused, "When I compare the time spent in psychiatry, pediatrics, surgery, obstetrics, geriatrics, medical and surgical nursing, plus other subjects, I wonder which student is more adequately trained? I believe the [college] student spreads herself too thin when she attempts to learn subjects remote from nursing."[33] Others complained that college nursing students were "sheltered" from patients and families, had "little actual contact with disease," and "depended too much on their instructors."[34]

Supporters of the hospital schools concluded that collegiate programs failed to adequately teach technical procedures. This, they argued, had a negative impact on the quality of bedside nursing care. Many expressed doubts, similar to those in Patricia Early's letter, about college graduates' ability to skillfully care for patients. One woman writing in 1960 complained that degreed nurses were "afraid to handle bedpans and give backrubs."[35] Two years later another critic, a hospital staff nurse, wrote, "If I am hospitalized, I hope that the nurses who care for me have a thorough education in nursing. I hope they know pharmacology, aseptic techniques, symptomology, and so on. I shall not care if they know a Van Gogh from a Rembrandt or have six credits in physical education."[36] This belief that

college programs produced nurses who knew more about Bach than back-rubs persisted well into the 1970s and 1980s. A letter published in 1977 illustrated this attitude as the author wondered, "How many mistakes [do] new graduates make that we never know about and how many procedures are bluffed through? What right have we to expose our patients to anything but clinically experienced nurses?"[37]

Nursing Science and Research

Nursing leaders, however, stated that the hospital schools did not offer the background needed for modern professional practice. As a Pennsylvania director of nursing observed, contemporary RNs needed coursework in "human relations, evaluation techniques, teaching skills, principles of supervision, community responsibility and participation, methods of research or approaches to the use of research findings."[38] Postwar college graduates likewise argued the need for a scientifically based training program. Two students wrote the following defense of degreed nurses in 1968: "In our opinion, the main objective of nursing is not to provide the patient with technical skills at the bedside, but to give individualized comprehensive nursing care that includes a complete understanding of the patient's physiological, emotional, sociological, and psychological needs. Thus, we feel that our collegiate background enables us to give this type of nursing care."[39]

Nursing leaders stressed that the college programs' emphasis on intellectual rather than manual skills resulted in superior learning experiences. In 1976, nurse-educator Rozella Scholtfeldt praised the university as the only place where students could learn important theories, engage in research, and benefit from the latest scientific findings.[40] Other collegiate faculty argued that learning theory enhanced patient care because students learned "the how and why of nursing procedures."[41] AJN editor Barbara Schutt suggested that colleges were more likely than hospitals to teach nursing students to think.[42]

College graduates, writing of their own experiences, also believed their faculty members were more likely than those in the hospital schools to give students freedom to inquire and experiment. This opportunity, they declared, improved their ability to make decisions, diagnose patients' needs, and facilitate change in a responsible manner.[43] One hospital staff nurse with a four-year degree explained that "when a patient questions the useful-

ness of a third I.V. that contains electrolytes, I can say more than 'the doctor ordered it' or 'it will make you feel better.' The academics help me to know why a patient fights back when a Levin tube is inserted so I can solve the problem on that level."[44]

Advocates of hospital education, however, were not reassured by these arguments. To hospital graduates schooled in a tradition of service, patient care was the sole reason for nursing's existence. They feared that the values of the university — theory, research, and intellectualism — fostered a false sense of superiority and led nurses on a quest for status at the expense of their patients. Responding to writers who praised the new scientific, theory-related educational programs, hospital graduates wondered whether their college-trained counterparts were interested in assuming the unglamorous work of patient care.[45] One nurse maintained that college-educated RNs were cold and unable to meet patients' emotional needs.[46] Another argued that college graduates were self-centered, concerned with "power, control, status, independence, money for me," not "commitment to and caring for others."[47] Still another concluded that college-trained nurses cared little about helping the sick and simply wanted "a Monday through Friday, 7–3 job."[48]

The Professionalism Debate

Some of the ire directed at college graduates came from fear. Hospital-trained RNs were alarmed by the leadership's second line of reasoning — that raising entry-level requirements attracted better qualified students. Although this rationale was similar to that advanced at the turn of the century, it lacked the earlier class bias. Post–World War II nursing leaders recognized that high school education had become almost universal and that college education was increasingly accessible. They maintained that the profession would not attract intelligent and competent high school graduates unless nursing followed accepted trends and moved its programs into higher education. In 1966, nursing educator Hildegard Peplau observed that "the widening middle class seeks [college] education, not training, for its able sons and daughters."[49] Almost ten years later, *AJN* editor Thelma Schorr echoed this line of reasoning. In a 1975 editorial, she urged rank-and-file nurses to accept the inevitable and support educational reform because "bright young men and women — the pool from which nursing must draw — are college-bound."[50]

College supporters also believed that raising the entry-level requirements ensured a professional identity for nurses, resulting in higher salaries
and an improved image. They argued that improvement would evolve only
when nurses, like professionals in other fields, held that all-important college degree. One woman, writing shortly after the ANA published its Position Paper, pointed out that teachers and physical therapists earned more
than nurses because their professions required a bachelor's degree.[51] Others
argued, as did an ADN graduate writing in 1976, that placing entry-level
education in colleges was "an excellent way of making nursing an acknowledged profession."[52] Still others believed that since colleges encouraged
inquiry, initiative, and experimentation rather than sheer obedience to
duty, moving educational programs to the university was a way to correct
the "master-servant relationship" between medicine and nursing and erase
the "handmaiden image" associated with RNs.[53]

Hospital-trained RNs, however, argued that their schools fostered
professionalism as well as colleges and universities did. Others suggested
that professionalism depended on individual qualifications rather than on
the type of school one attended.[54] Hospital graduates bridled at the sugges-
tion that they were less professional than their college-educated coworkers.
As one pointed out in 1966, "Diploma school graduates take the same state
board examinations, pay the same [license] fees, and even pay the same
ANA dues [as the college graduates]."[55] To many nurses the distinctions
between the ADN, BSN, and hospital school diploma seemed fuzzy and
artificial. A clinical specialist voiced these frustrations in a 1979 letter:

> I have become certified in my specialty; I am active in continuing education. I
> have been active on committees in local and state professional organizations.
> I have leadership, planning, organizing, psych-social-bio and technical skills. I
> am not able to discern in what areas I do not qualify as a professional nurse.
> Is it really all explained by those three letters — BSN? Perhaps the main reason
> I am not a professional in spite of my experience, abilities, and status is that I
> don't understand what I'm lacking in professionalism.[56]

Because of this growing association of a college degree with professionalism, hospital graduates believed mandatory entry-level college degrees would hurt them. Particularly after 1966, numerous letters and articles
appeared in the professional press pondering the effect educational reform
would have on salaries and promotion opportunities. Nurses argued that
hospital graduates would experience discrimination. Several feared employers would hire and promote only those with college degrees.[57] Another

wondered how nurses' personal mobility would be affected as they moved between states in various stages of licensure change.[58] To hospital graduates it seemed as though their own profession had conspired against them. Changing educational requirements had deprofessionalized them and devalued their skills and dedication. Most of all, they felt expendable. It seemed as though the professional associations, nursing leaders, and their younger, college-educated colleagues had changed the rules in midstream without thought of the consequences to RNs trained in an apprenticeship tradition. A hospital nursing administrator from Los Angeles described a conversation with two head nurses in 1966 that captured the sense of betrayal felt by hospital-educated RNs: "Here they were: competent, capable, dedicated, hardworking, intelligent, *caring* women. They *chose* these schools not because they couldn't go to college, but because this was the kind of program *they* wanted. They *were* proud to be registered nurses, proud of their contributions, proud of their profession, but in their own minds, they have been 'cast out.'" [Emphasis in original.][59]

Thus, the conflict over educational reform continued as nurses battled over the entry-into-practice issue. Nursing leaders and college-trained RNs believed professional education should include theoretical knowledge, be scientifically grounded, and prepare nurses to think and practice independently. They also saw educational reform as a way of recruiting the best qualified American students and as an important step in upgrading nursing's salaries and status.

Rank-and-file hospital graduates saw the issue differently. They were noticeably less inclined to support the educational reform. Their beliefs about professional training conflicted with those of both the leadership and the younger, college-educated nurses. They perceived nursing as an occupation that required technical, hands-on expertise and dedication to serving the patient. They feared new trends would jeopardize quality care.

Hospital graduates also objected to educational reform because they believed the association of "professional" with "college-educated" endangered their own careers. Since the opposing camps approached the issue with such distinct beliefs, adversaries found it difficult to understand each other's point of view. Given the potential of this issue to affect nurses' earnings, career possibilities, status, and autonomy, neither side was inclined to compromise. Despite changes in health care delivery, public support for higher education, and new arguments from nursing leaders, entry-into-practice was as divisive in the post–World War II era as it had been half a century earlier.

SUSAN RIMBY LEIGHOW, PHD
History Department
Shippensburg University
1871 Old Main Drive
Shippensburg, Pa. 17257
Phone: (717)532-1265

Acknowledgments

The author would like to thank the staff members of the National League for Nursing and the Pennsylvania Nurses Association for their assistance.

Notes

1. Patricia Early, "Letters," *American Journal of Nursing* 66 (April 1966): 738 (hereafter cited as *AJN*).
2. See Susan Armeny, "Resolute Enthusiasts: The Effort to Professionalize American Nursing, 1880–1915" (PhD diss., University of Missouri-Columbia, 1983), 157–95, 278–97, 398–99; Barbara Melosh, *"The Physician's Hand": Work Culture and Conflict in American Nursing* (Philadelphia: Temple University Press, 1982), 3–5, 30–34, 40–44, 123–24; and Susan M. Reverby, *Ordered to Care: The Dilemma of American Nursing, 1850–1945* (New York: Cambridge University Press, 1987), 97–99, 121–42, 159–77.
3. Before World War II, only a handful of collegiate programs were established. These catered to licensed nurses seeking advanced degrees. For an analysis of the failure of educational reform prior to World War II, see Armeny, 278–97; Melosh, 27–28; and Reverby, 164–73.
4. See Shirley H. Fondiller, *The Entry Dilemma: The National League for Nursing and the Higher Education Movement, 1952–1972, With an Epilogue to 1983* (New York: NLN, 1980); Melosh, 68–69; and Reverby, 203.
5. ANA, *Facts About Nursing, 1951* (New York: ANA, 1951), 51.
6. See JoAnn Ashley, *Hospitals, Paternalism and the Role of the Nurse* (New York: Teachers College Press, 1976); Philip A. Kalisch and Beatrice J. Kalisch, *The Advance of American Nursing,* 2nd ed. (Boston: Little, Brown, and Company, 1986), 101–23, 161–94; Melosh, 47–67; Reverby, 60–75; and Nancy Tomes, "Little World of Our Own," in *Women and Health in America,* ed. Judith Walzer Leavitt (Madison: University of Wisconsin Press, 1984), 470.
7. See Melosh, 40–41; and Reverby, 170–76.
8. See ANA, *Facts About Nursing, 1955–56* (New York: ANA, 1956), 190; ANA, *Facts About Nursing, 1964* (New York: ANA, 1964), 244, 247; and ANA, *Facts About Nursing, 1968* (New York: ANA, 1968), 222, 224, 227.
9. See Zella Bryant and Helen V. Hudson, "The Census of Nurses in Public

Health," *AJN* 62 (December 1962): 104; Vera Freeman, "Staff Nurse Vacancies in Selected Public Health Nursing Agencies — 1961," *Nursing Outlook* 10 (February 1962): 112; Mildred Gaynor, "Public Health Nursing for the Future," *Nursing Outlook* 5 (July 1957): 399; and "News Highlights," *AJN* 58 (April 1958): 494.

10. See Clara A. Hardin, "Supply of Professional Nurses in 1956," *AJN* 56 (December 1956): 1546; and Roberta R. Spohn, "Some Facts About the Nursing Shortage," *AJN* 54 (July 1954): 865–67.

11. Kalisch and Kalisch, 575–92.

12. See "AMA Issues Statement on Resuscitation by R.N.'s," *AJN* 68 (February 1968): 2; and Barbara G. Schutt, "More Than Two Hands," *AJN* 68 (February 1968): 43.

13. Melosh, 190.

14. See Bonnie Bullough, "Influences in Role Expansion," *AJN* 76 (September 1976): 1478–79; Melosh, 197; Evelyn Moses and Aleda Roth, "Nursepower: What Do Statistics Reveal About the Nation's Nurses?" *AJN* 79 (October 1979): 1753; and Reverby, 203.

15. See Burton Bledstein, *The Culture of Professionalism: The Middle Class and the Development of Higher Education in America* (New York: W. W. Norton and Company, 1976), 293; and Harold S. Wechsler, *The Qualified Student: A History of Selective College Admissions in America* (New York: John Wiley and Sons, 1977), 3–12.

16. See Ernest L. Boyer and Arthur Levine, *A Quest for Common Learning: The Aims of General Education* (Washington, D.C.: The Carnegie Foundation for the Advancement of Teaching, n.d.), 21; Marcia Graham Synott, *The Half-Opened Door: Discrimination and Admissions at Harvard, Yale, and Princeton, 1900–1970* (Westport, Conn.: Greenwood Press, 1979), 199–201; and Wechsler, 251–54.

17. Wechsler, 259–60.

18. Armeny, 300.

19. See Esther Lucille Brown, "Professional Education for the Nursing of the Future," *AJN* 47 (December 1947): 7; and Susan Rimby Leighow, " 'Nurses' Questions/Women's Questions': The Impact of the Demographic Revolution and Feminism on United States Working Women, 1946–1986" (PhD diss., University of Pittsburgh, 1992), 32–33.

20. See ANA, *Facts About Nursing, 1962–63* (New York: ANA, 1963), 102; Kalisch and Kalisch, 590, 644, 664; Edith S. Oshin, "How to Get Help for Your Education," *RN* 24 (November 1961): 44–51; M. Gale Rubenfeld et al., "The Nurse Training Act: Yesterday, Today, and . . . ," *AJN* 81 (June 1981): 1202; and Jessie M. Scott, "Federal Support for Nursing Education, 1964 to 1972," *AJN* 72 (October 1972): 1857–58.

21. See Kalisch and Kalisch, 698; and Beatrice M. Shriver et al., "Follow-up on Mental Health Trainees," *AJN* 67 (December 1967): 2572.

22. See Georgeen H. DeChow, "The Development of an Associate Degree Nursing Program," *Journal of Nursing Education* 1 (September 1962): 35–36; Mildred L. Montag, "Technical Eduction in Nursing?" *AJN* 63 (May 1963): 100–103; and Rosemarie Rizzo Parse, "The Advantages of the Associate Degree Program," *Journal of Nursing Education* 6 (August 1967): 17.

23. "One Resolution Is Revised at Final Business Meeting," *NLN News* (n.d.), NLN Headquarters, New York City, 13. See also "Resolutions Voted Friday," *NLN News* (n.d.), NLN Headquarters, New York City, 13.

24. ANA, "Education for Nursing," *AJN* 65 (December 1965): 107–8.

25. See Fondiller, 58–68, 95–100, 116–17; and Kalisch and Kalisch, 564–65.

26. See "ANA Delegates Vote to Limit RN Title to BSN Grad," *AJN* 85 (September 1985): 1016, 1020; "National League for Nursing Convention," *Nursing Outlook* 15 (June 1967): 54; "NJSNA Withdraws Support of BSN for Entry into Practice," *Nursing Outlook* 28 (January 1980): 15; "NLN Board Endorses BSN for Professional Practice," *Nursing Outlook* 30 (April 1982): 217; and "NLN Reaffirms Its BSN Stance Despite 'Technical Nursing' Rift," *AJN* 83 (July 1983): 985, 994.

27. See Lucie S. Kelly, "A Little Game of Russian Roulette," *Nursing Outlook* 34 (May/June 1986): 123; Lucie S. Kelly, "New Titles for Nurses: Prelude to What?" *Nursing Outlook* 34 (May/June 1986): 120; and Elizabeth A. Waidowicz, "Letters," *Nursing Outlook* 33 (May 1985): 254.

28. See Fondiller, 116; and Kelly, "New Titles for Nurses," 120.

29. See Delna M. Day, "Letters," *AJN* 71 (March 1971): 486; Mabel M. Linkous, "Letters," *AJN* 67 (July 1967): 1410; Joy S. Mead, "Letters," *AJN* 68 (February 1968): 269; and E. Charlotte Theis, "Our Readers Say," *Nursing Outlook* 27 (July 1979): 439.

30. Annabel C. Taltavull, "Our Readers Say," *Nursing Outlook* 14 (July 1966): 23.

31. Vivian M. Keeney, "Letters," *AJN* 69 (July 1969): 1430.

32. Barbara Lagoon, "Letters," *AJN* 67 (February 1967): 262.

33. Hazel Head, "Letters," *AJN* 67 (September 1967): 1829.

34. Margaret S. Brown, "Letters," *AJN* 67 (October 1967): 2058; Vivian J. Cummings, "Letters," *AJN* 78 (January 1978): 24; Jean G. French, "About Community Nursing in the Future," *Nursing Outlook* 19 (March 1971): 175.

35. Evelyn Hardy, "Letters," *AJN* 60 (December 1960): 1702.

36. R. Meyer, "Letters," *AJN* 62 (August 1962): 16.

37. Bonnie L. Clark, "Letters," *AJN* 77 (August 1977): 1279.

38. Rita Sinkevitch, "A Director of Nursing Speaks on Education," *The Pennsylvania Nurse* 22 (January 1967): 7.

39. Kay Johnston and Diane Jensen, "Letters," *AJN* 68 (June 1968): 1212.

40. Rozella Scholtfeldt, "Rozella Scholtfeldt Says . . . ," *AJN* 76 (January 1976): 107.

41. Laura C. Dustan, "Education for Nursing: Apprenticeship or Academic," *Nursing Outlook* 15 (September 1967): 30. See also Margaret McClure, "Margaret McClure Says . . . ," *AJN* 76 (January 1976): 102.

42. Barbara G. Schutt, "The Free Mind," *AJN* 67 (January 1967): 57.

43. See Johnston and Jensen, 1212; and Yvonne Kemp, "Our Readers Say," *Nursing Outlook* 23 (September 1975): 538.

44. Nancy Carothers, "Letters," *AJN* 68 (October 1968): 2115.

45. See Shirley Holt, "Our Readers Say," *Nursing Outlook* 24 (July 1976): 468; and Jean Linn, "Letters," *AJN* 80 (February 1980): 224.

46. Joan N. Robinson, "Letters," *AJN* 78 (November 1978): 1871.

47. Claudia Appeldorn, "Our Readers Say," *Nursing Outlook* 27 (August 1979): 501.

48. Connie Richardson, "Letters," *AJN* 78 (October 1978): 1656.

49. Hildegard E. Peplau, "Our Readers Say," *Nursing Outlook* 14 (August 1966): 22.

50. Thelma M. Schorr, "The New York Plan," *AJN* 75 (December 1975): 2141.

51. Marilyn J. Henning, "Letters," *AJN* 66 (November 1966): 2404.

52. Nancy Divistea, "Letters," *AJN* 76 (August 1976): 1250.

53. Nancy Carothers, "Letters," *AJN* 68 (October 1968): 2115; Joan Livesay, "Letters," *AJN* 79 (April 1979): 620.

54. See Jacqueline Childers, "Letters," *AJN* 66 (April 1966): 734; Dawn Hoosier, "Our Readers Say," *Nursing Outlook* 34 (January/February 1986): 8; Michele A. Luna, "Our Readers Say," *Nursing Outlook* 26 (July 1978): 408; Victoria Mehr, "Our Readers Say," *Nursing Outlook* 28 (May 1980): 272; Patricia Offer, "Letters," *AJN* 77 (March 1977): 394, 396; and Patricia B. Perry, "Our Readers Say," *Nursing Outlook* 30 (June 1982): 327.

55. R.N., "Letters," *AJN* 66 (May 1966): 995.

56. Suzanne D. Schutze, "Letters," *AJN* 79 (September 1979): 1540.

57. See Janice Armstrong, "Letters," *AJN* 79 (October 1979): 1710; Kathleen E. Benedette, "Letters," *AJN* 68 (February 1968): 279; Laura Erdel, "Letters," *AJN* 79 (June 1979): 1057; and Helen G. Wolford, "Letters," *AJN* 79 (May 1979): 880.

58. Erline P. McGriff, "Two New York Nurses Debate the NYSNA 1985 Proposal," *AJN* 76 (June 1976): 932.

59. Evelyn M. Hamil, "What Good Is Reason When Dreams Are Shattered?" *AJN* 66 (June 1966): 1344.

The Historical Relationship of Nursing Program Accreditation and Public Policy in Canada

SHARON L. RICHARDSON
Faculty of Nursing
University of Alberta

In North America, accreditation of nursing education programs has been promoted as a mechanism for ensuring that predetermined standards are met. The National League for Nursing (NLN) is the accrediting agency in the United States, and the Canadian Association of University Schools of Nursing (CAUSN) sponsors a voluntary accreditation program for university schools of nursing in Canada. Acceptance of accreditation has been greater in the United States than in Canada. Unlike the situation in the United States, only one-third of Canada's 33 baccalaureate programs are currently accredited, and there is no accreditation available for the 122 diploma programs that continue to prepare three-quarters of all Canadian nurses to enter practice, or for the 13 graduate programs that prepare advanced practitioners, teachers, and administrators. In comparison, in the United States a significant majority of diploma, associate degree, baccalaureate, and master's programs are accredited by the NLN.

The purpose of my research was to analyze the history of nursing education program accreditation in Canada within the context of public policy and to contrast it with the history of American nursing education accreditation. Accreditation is defined as a voluntary process involving national standards established to improve educational programming and the quality of graduates.[1] A distinction is made in Canada between *accreditation* and *approval* of nursing education programs. Approval is a mandatory process involving minimum standards established provincially by regulating agencies to ensure safe graduates, whereas accreditation is a voluntary process involving national standards established by nongovernmental organizations to promote high-quality educational programming and exemplary

Nursing History Review 4 (1996): 19–41. Copyright © 1996 by The American Association for the History of Nursing.

graduates.² Public policy is a long series of more or less related choices, including decisions not to act, which are made by governments in response to public issues.³

History of Canadian Nursing Program Accreditation

In Canada, as in the United States, nursing leaders initially promoted accreditation of nursing education programs as a way to bring about improvements in hospital schools.

EARLY NURSING EDUCATION
Since the first program to train nurses was instituted at the General and Marine Hospital in St. Catherines, Ontario, in 1874, education of nurses for entry to practice in Canada has been inextricably interwoven with the development of hospitals. Largely philanthropic in purpose, early training schools did not differentiate between the goals of providing nursing service for the hospital and that of developing a good educational system in the school.⁴ As hospitals increased in number, it soon became an almost universally accepted principle that a school of nursing was indispensable in the operation of the hospital. Student nurses constituted the majority of nursing service department workers, and the hospital's need for nursing service dictated the number and characteristics of individuals admitted for training. These hospital programs have been described erroneously as apprenticeships, despite the fact that for many years students learned on the job by working in the wards, often without supervision or previous instruction. Unlike Nightingale's famous model established in conjunction with St. Thomas' Hospital, London, these schools were neither financially nor organizationally independent of the sponsoring hospital.

Until the Second World War, the majority of hospital school graduates practiced as private duty nurses and contracted their services to individuals and families in the community and, less frequently, in hospitals. Only a limited number of graduate nurses were employed by hospitals, and they functioned in supervisory positions to oversee the nursing work done by students. Few graduate nurses were hired to provide direct patient care in what became known as general duty or staff nurse roles. Early in the twentieth century, it was also common practice for hospitals to send the more experienced student nurses into clients' homes and to use the fees thus collected to offset operating costs of the hospital. The students received

none of this remuneration. This hospital practice further reduced employ-ment options for graduate nurses.

Limited standards for hospital schools of nursing existed prior to the Second World War. Usually, some standards were contained in the provin-cial nursing registration acts, which were in place in all provinces by 1922; however, these standards were both rudimentary in nature and infrequently enforced. As noted by Weir in the 1930 *Survey of Nursing Education in Canada:*

> At the present time, in the majority of provinces, practically any person operat-ing a hospital can establish in connection therewith a training school for stu-dent nurses. While the school may be approved, there is at present no legal barrier to its creation or to its graduates posing as qualified nurses. In a num-ber of cases brought to the attention of the Survey, these alleged schools are little more than economic annexes designed for the supply of cheap hospital labour. Their pretence at offering an educational course of training should be considered little other than a mere sham.[5]

Many Canadian hospital training programs of the 1920s, 1930s, and 1940s were characterized by limited coordination of classroom and bedside teaching, long hours, much night duty without supervision, and many housekeeping tasks. Clinical experience was limited if the hospital was small, and teaching by the medical staff and the few nursing supervisors was haphazard and poorly planned.[6]

Weir made a number of specific recommendations to improve hospital training programs and advocated the development of training schools for nurses primarily as educational institutions, functioning as an integral part of the general education system of the province and financed on the same principle as the teacher training schools.[7] This latter recommendation echoed that of the 1914 Special Committee on Nurse Education, headed by President Falconer of the University of Toronto, that training schools be separated from hospitals to permit significant improvement in the educa-tion offered to student nurses.[8]

PUBLIC POLICY
Despite the obvious problems in hospital training programs illuminated by the Weir report and the gradual expansion of hospitals that followed the First World War, no action was taken by provincial governments to require hospitals to address inadequate student admission criteria, poor programs of instruction, overwork of students, and oversupply of graduates. Under

the 1867 British North America Act, both health and education fell within provincial rather than national jurisdiction. There were several reasons for provincial inaction. First and probably foremost, the development of hospitals and their training schools had followed a pattern of voluntarism in control and financing, which meant that hospitals were essentially autonomous in their operations because they received limited revenue from the provinces and operated philanthropically.[9] Therefore, provincial departments of health and education had limited influence over the organization and operation of hospital-sponsored nursing programs.

Because both health and education fell under provincial and not federal jurisdiction, there was little the federal government could do directly to influence changes in nursing education. Federal-provincial government relations historically have been at issue in the formulation of public policy in Canada. The national party in power and its prime minister have been careful not to antagonize provincial governments by intruding into matters clearly within provincial jurisdiction. Hospital nurse training was one of the few occupations open to women before the Second World War, along with teaching and secretarial work. As long as hospitals were able to recruit sufficient students to staff their units, there was little impetus for change. In exchange for work, student nurses received free on-the-job training and the possibility of self-employment at the end of the training program. From the hospitals' perspective, this was a fair exchange. From the provincial governments' perspectives, there was no need to fix something that was not broken, and from the federal government's perspective, there were other national issues with higher priority than improving the education of a relatively small portion of the Canadian labor force.

Not unexpectedly, opposition to the improvements in hospital training programs, such as those indicated in the Weir report, was concentrated among hospital superintendents and, to a lesser extent, physicians.[10] Hospital superintendents feared the financial cost that might result from replacing unsalaried student workers with salaried graduate nurses. The cost of providing nursing education was taken for granted as being offset by salary savings associated with student service, even though there was little factual information to support this belief and no research evidence. Physicians expressed concern that graduate nurses would usurp the role of medical staff.

The Great Depression also delayed reform in hospital training programs. Because hospitals provided training and room and board free of charge in exchange for student service, there was no dearth of applicants. Hospitals also benefited from hiring graduate nurses who were unable to

find private duty employment because clients could not pay for their services. These graduates were often willing to provide full-time service to hospitals in exchange for room and board and a few dollars a month.[11] Their service further reduced the number of students needed, contributing to smaller school enrollments and limiting the perceived need for improvement in educational programming.

The organized nursing profession itself was unable to significantly influence formulation of public policy affecting either nursing work or education. The emerging provincial nursing associations lacked sufficient membership, personnel, and fiscal resources to lobby effectively for improved hospital training programs. Not until 1922 did all nine provincial nurses' associations have some form of nurse registration legislation on which to base nursing education standards.[12] Even then, the process of approving schools of nursing based on predetermined standards was a hit-and-miss activity in most provinces and nonexistent in some. Additionally, nurse registration was voluntary, and the provincial nursing associations tended to be small, with limited personnel, expertise, and money. The Canadian Nurses Association (CNA), a federation of provincial nursing associations, formed in 1924, which were self-governing units free to accept or reject the advice offered by the national association, could act only in an advisory capacity. This it sought to do, first, through cosponsorship with the Canadian Medical Association of the 1932 *Survey of Nursing Education in Canada* (for which it bore 70 percent of the overall costs), and later through formulation and publication in 1936 of *A Proposed Curriculum for Schools of Nursing*. Adoption of the *Proposed Curriculum* was voluntary in schools of nursing, thus limiting its impact.

Because of the constraints associated with the autonomy of hospitals that operated schools of nursing and the lack of effective regulations governing their educational programs, the system of hospital nurse training established by the beginning of the twentieth century in Canada remained essentially unchanged until the upheaval of the Second World War.

Impact of the Second World War

The Second World War and its immediate aftermath had a considerable impact on both nursing work and nursing education in Canada. The most immediate effect was the extreme shortage of nurses when 4,000 graduates entered direct wartime service.[13] Existing inadequacies in hospital training

were highlighted when the number of applicants declined dramatically as young women took advantage of a wider variety of appealing career options. The shortage of qualified high school graduates willing to endure the three-year training program and the abandonment of hospital nursing by graduates for other occupations with better employment conditions and remuneration continued after the war.[14] Long hours of work, excessive housekeeping duties, unreasonable workloads, and poor levels of pay in most hospitals caused many graduate nurses to enter branches of nursing with better employment conditions or to leave nursing altogether. In 1946, the CNA estimated the shortage of nurses in hospitals to be 7,000.[15] Many Canadian graduate nurses, especially those with experience and postgraduate credentials, were attracted to the United States, where salaries were considerably higher.

As part of a program to alleviate the severe wartime shortage of graduate and student nurses, the federal government provided funds for nursing education that were administered through the CNA.[16] Although these funds eased some immediate problems, they did not lead to any significant change in the system of education, which remained predominantly hospital-controlled on-the-job training. These funds did, however, provide the CNA with sufficient financial support at a crucial time in its corporate development, enabling it to significantly expand its role and activities.[17] The federal grants of 1942 through 1948 permitted the CNA to consolidate its position as the national nursing association in Canada, speaking on behalf of organized nursing. Soon after the Second World War, the CNA became more active in public policy affecting both nursing education and nursing work.

THE CNA AND ACCREDITATION

The concept of accreditation as a specific strategy to improve hospital training first surfaced at the 1944 Annual General Meeting of the CNA.[18] The following year, the CNA approved the principle of accreditation and directed a committee to initiate a plan of action as soon as possible.[19] However, the committee's subsequent plan was tabled by the executive in 1946 because of limited funds and other, more urgent projects.[20] From 1946 through 1952, the CNA was extensively involved with the Canadian Red Cross in a demonstration school of nursing that was independent of hospital control and prepared students in two rather than three years.[21] The success of this demonstration school, which was affiliated with the Metro-

politan General Hospital in Windsor, Ontario, paved the way in Canada for two-year diploma nursing programs independent of hospitals.

ACCREDITATION PILOT PROJECT

In the mid-1950s, stimulated by a program of evaluation of schools of nursing developed by the Canadian Conference of Catholic Schools of Nursing[22] and the successful unification of nursing program accreditation under the NLN in the United States, the CNA determined to "undertake without delay steps leading toward a program for the accreditation of schools of nursing; . . . and to conduct a pilot study involving as many schools in as many regions as possible."[23] A project director was hired and the assistance of the NLN was sought to conduct the pilot study whose purpose was "[t]o determine if Canadian schools of nursing are ready for a program of accreditation, and if it is feasible at this time to initiate such a program."[24] The actual pilot study, lasting from 1957 to 1959, involved assessing 25 of Canada's 171 hospital schools using criteria, tools, and procedures developed by the American NLN. From a list of volunteer schools, 25 schools were selected to provide a range of large and small, urban and rural, lay and religiously affiliated schools from across the country.

The success of the pilot project was substantially limited by its principal conclusion "that Canadian schools of nursing as a whole are not ready for a program of accreditation . . . [and] on the basis of the over-all quality . . . only 16 per cent of these schools would merit accreditation."[25] Only 4 of the 25 participating hospital schools evaluated were adjudged to merit accreditation using the American standards. Arguably, this outcome seriously impeded further CNA accreditation activities. Commitment to the concept of accreditation as a way of assisting hospital schools to enhance their educational programs waned and enthusiasm among CNA membership for a national program of accreditation was limited during the years following the publication of the pilot project report. During the ensuing two decades, the CNA executive struggled unsuccessfully to develop a national program of accreditation for hospital schools, and a series of ad hoc committees that were struck to examine accreditation foundered.[26] An attempt in the late 1970s to collaborate with the CAUSN, which was developing a program of voluntary accreditation for baccalaureate programs, came to naught when the Kellogg Foundation declined funding.[27] Subsequent attempts by the CNA to locate external funding were unsuccessful.[28] In 1982, the CNA ceased all activities associated with accreditation.[29]

PUBLIC POLICY

Hospital nurse educators' disillusionment with accreditation as a strategy to enhance programming led them to fall back on provincial approval. Following the Second World War, Canadian provincial nursing associations had considerable input, if not control, over standards affecting diploma nursing programs. In six provinces — British Columbia, Saskatchewan, Manitoba, New Brunswick, Nova Scotia, and Newfoundland — the provincial nursing associations, in addition to controlling nurse registration, had been delegated the responsibility for defining and monitoring minimum standards for approval of schools of nursing.[30] In Ontario, Quebec, and Alberta, the educational ministry or an appointed committee approved diploma schools of nursing. In each of the latter three provinces, the provincial nursing association had input into setting and revising standards through consultation and/or representation on the committee.[31] Thus, the national appeal of accreditation was attenuated by provincial nursing associations' control or significant influence over the approval of diploma programs.

Long-awaited changes in diploma nursing education in the 1960s and 1970s also defused concern about the need for accreditation as a strategy to bring about reform. Heeding the recommendations of the 1964 Royal Commission on Health Services — and spurred on by the increased demand for nursing service after the federal government's 1948 National Health Grants Programs triggered massive hospital construction — Ontario, Quebec, and Saskatchewan began in the late 1960s to transfer diploma nursing education from the control of hospitals into the province's general education system. This transfer was facilitated in Ontario and Quebec by the creation and rapid growth of community colleges. Community college programs were two years in length and resulted in an increase in the number of graduates entering practice in two-thirds of the time required by hospital training schools. This was because hospital training programs continued to be three years in length so that students could repay the cost of their training in service. College nursing students paid tuition and had no service requirements. The educational soundness of two-year diploma nursing programs had been demonstrated repeatedly in Ontario by pilot projects conducted during the 1950s.[32] The 1964 Royal Commission on Health Services had recommended diploma programs of less than three years' duration which functioned independently from hospitals because "[t]he educational system for nursing should be organized and financed like other forms of professional education [and] . . . not only shall we obtain equally,

if not better, qualified personnel in shorter time, but a substantial part of hospitalized patient-care will no longer depend . . . upon apprentices."[33]

Another outcome of the 1964 Royal Commission on Health Services was the provincial governments' renewed interest in evaluating schools of nursing. Because of the increased role of the provincial ministries of health in the regulation of hospitals' and physicians' services (resulting from the implementation of universal hospital insurance in the late 1950s and universal medical insurance in the late 1960s), it became possible to strengthen the mechanisms for approving nursing schools in an attempt to standardize programs and ensure that minimum criteria were met. Hospitals, too, came increasingly under the scrutiny and control of provincial ministries of health, allowing the formulation of public policy affecting hospital nurse training programs.

By 1975, hospital training schools had been phased out completely in Saskatchewan, Ontario, and Quebec, and independent schools had been established in New Brunswick, which had no community colleges.[34] Community college programs were initiated in Alberta and British Columbia during the 1960s and 1970s, although no hospital programs were closed.[35] Opposition from the Canadian Hospital Association and its provincial affiliates, who feared losing control over nurse training programs and losing student services, effectively stalled total transfer of diploma nursing education into the postsecondary educational systems of Newfoundland, Prince Edward Island, Nova Scotia, Manitoba, Alberta, and British Columbia.[36] In his history of Canadian hospitals, Harvey Agnew likened the Canadian Hospital Association's viewpoint on hospital training schools to that of the medical profession a decade earlier regarding national health insurance, asserting that it was "compounded of the unknown."[37] Nonetheless, a decade after the 1964 Report of the Royal Commission on Health Services, more than three-quarters of all Canadian diploma nurses graduated from programs in the general education systems of the provinces.[38]

Accreditation of University Programs

Accreditation of university nursing programs took an entirely different course from that of diploma programs in Canada. In part this was because university nursing education grew slowly in Canada, although programs to prepare public health nurses were financed by the Red Cross as early as the 1920s at the Universities of Toronto, McGill, British Columbia, Alberta,

and Dalhousie.[39] Early university nursing education consisted mainly of certificate courses for graduates of the hospital training schools, which prepared them for positions in public health and, later, teaching and administration. Before the Second World War, small baccalaureate programs preparing a limited number of graduate nurses had been established at the Universities of British Columbia, Alberta, Saskatchewan, Western Ontario, and Ottawa and the Institut Marguerite d'Youville (affiliated with the University of Montreal).[40] In addition, diploma, but not degree, programs had been initiated at McGill University[41] and the University of Toronto.[42] The small size of these and subsequent programs is attested to by the fact that, as late as 1962, less than 4 percent of all students enrolled in nursing education geared toward entry into practice were attending universities.[43]

The growth of university schools of nursing was greatest during the 1960s, when several new schools opened and existing schools expanded. Financial and teaching resources were redirected to baccalaureate programs from certificate programming, and the first master's programs in nursing were begun to prepare teachers and administrators.[44] Although the CAUSN had published *Desirable General Standards for Canadian University Schools of Nursing* in 1957, there were few formal standards for baccalaureate programs and limited provincial government approval mechanisms. The CAUSN itself was a fledgling organization composed of a loose affiliation of individual university nurse educators that met once or twice a year nationally and once or twice regionally. It had few resources, no secretariat, and minimal influence on university nursing education before its restructuring in 1967. The tendency in Canadian university nursing education was toward individual program evaluation as part of universities' normal academic activity.

CAUSN Involvement in Accreditation

The issue of accreditation for university nursing programs surfaced in 1971 at the National Conference on Assistance to the Physician, when the federal minister of health recommended the creation of a national body to accredit all health disciplines.[45] Although not opposed to some kind of national program of accreditation, university nursing deans did not support government control, because they feared accreditation based on minimum standards would maintain the status quo and stymie progress.[46] Acting in concert, at the fall 1972 meeting of the recently restructured CAUSN, the deans unanimously declared "[t]hat CAUSN assume responsibility for the accreditting [*sic*] function for university schools of nursing and be recognized

as an accreditting [*sic*] agency."[47] Establishing standards for university nursing programs had been a stated goal of the CAUSN since its inception in 1942, and the deans clearly perceived university program accreditation as their prerogative.

Over the next fourteen years, the CAUSN devoted much of its time, energy, and resources to developing a national program of voluntary accreditation for baccalaureate nursing education. An appointed ad hoc committee of nondean nurse academics selected criteria, developed standards, created assessment tools and procedures, and drafted orientation documents for program appraisers. With the exception of a $5,000 grant received in 1976 from the Canadian Nurses Foundation, the CAUSN bore the entire cost of developing the national accreditation program. Membership fees were increased dramatically in 1978 to finance the accreditation program,[48] and the $100,200 reserve that had been created by fall 1981 proved essential to its implementation.[49]

Resistance to government involvement in accreditation of educational programs, particularly for physicians, coupled with the perception that the federal government's proposed coordinating agency was too large and unwieldy, led in 1976 to the withdrawal of the federal proposal, but the CAUSN did not abandon its accreditation program. The Ontario region of the CAUSN was especially anxious to have in place an accreditation program that could be used in lieu of the approval process developed to evaluate community college diploma nursing programs. At each stage in the development of the accreditation program, approval was sought from the CAUSN council, so that when the entire package was presented for final endorsement in 1986 by the deans, there were no surprises. The CAUSN council approved the ad hoc committee's proposal, and the first baccalaureate program to request and receive accreditation was at the University of Montreal in 1987. Over the next five years, ten reviews were completed, and a number of other baccalaureate programs were placed on a waiting list.[50]

Summary of Canadian Nursing Program Accreditation History

Accreditation of Canadian nursing programs was initially impeded by the publication in 1960 of the CNA's *Report of the Pilot Project for the Evaluation of Schools of Nursing in Canada,* which concluded that hospital schools were not ready for a program of accreditation because only 16 percent would

merit accreditation if such a program existed. This report disillusioned nurse educators who were already ambivalent about the benefits of accreditation, and it contributed to the CNA's eventual inability to sustain membership interest in a national accreditation program. Further interest in diploma program accreditation was constrained when provincial governments began to restructure nursing education in the 1960s and 1970s by transferring diploma programs from hospital control into provincial systems of postsecondary education. Provincial governments' assumption of responsibility for the education of health professionals coincided with their increased involvement in health care policy, particularly in the implementation of universal hospital insurance in the late 1950s and universal medical insurance in the late 1960s.[51]

University schools of nursing initiated a national program of voluntary accreditation through the CAUSN in accordance with the federal government's 1971 desire to establish accreditation for all health disciplines. Following the withdrawal of the federal proposal in 1976, the CAUSN continued to develop an accreditation program as a way of helping member schools upgrade their programming. The CAUSN's accreditation program was successfully implemented in 1986, and since that date it has accredited about one-third of all thirty-three Canadian baccalaureate nursing programs. In recent years, some university schools have resisted evaluation of their programs using minimum standards by negotiating substitution of accreditation for approval in provinces where agencies outside the universities appraise the baccalaureate programs. As more diploma nursing programs are phased out and the remaining programs enter into collaborations with universities, there is potential that the CAUSN's accreditation program will expand.

Brief History of American Nursing Program Accreditation

The history of nursing program accreditation in the United States is both more extensive and more complex than in Canada. A succinct history of American nursing program accreditation was offered by Helen Nahm in a June 1974 speech to the CAUSN in Toronto, Ontario.[52] Nahm asserted, "In a sense the development of accrediting programs in nursing [in the United States] could be looked upon as a last resort of nurse leaders to bring about improvements in nursing and nursing education after all other methods had failed."[53] Failed methods included fact-finding studies, such as those by

the Rockefeller Foundation in the early 1920s and the Grading Committee Studies of 1926 to 1934; distribution of curriculum guides; cost studies; and publication of facts about admissions, graduations, and withdrawals of students. Nahm stated that although "many improvements in nursing education programs were made during the 1930's, they were not of a magnitude sufficient to correct the inequities that had developed over a long period of years."[54]

At the end of the Second World War, Dr. Esther Lucile Brown was commissioned by the National Nursing Council to study nursing education in the United States. Her report, *Nursing for the Future,* was a catalyst toward further study by the National Committee for the Improvement of Nursing Services, an ad hoc committee struck by the joint board of the six national nursing organizations. The National Committee collected questionnaire data from 97 percent of all state-approved schools of nursing in the United States in 1949. These data were subjected to statistical analysis, and schools were then ranked according to certain agreed-upon criteria relating to curricula, faculty preparation, student welfare, and finances.[55] The top 25 percent were classified as Group I schools, the middle 50 percent as Group II schools, and the lowest 25 percent as Group III schools. Lists of Group I and Group II schools were published in the October 1949 issue of the *American Journal of Nursing.*[56] This created a furor in American nursing, which Nahn described as comparable only to that which followed publication in 1948 of the Brown Report.[57]

To propitiate critics when the 1949 classification was published, the National Committee promised the schools of nursing that a second or follow-up study would be conducted within two years. The National Nursing Accrediting Service, which had come into being on 1 January 1949,[58] was asked to conduct this second study. It coordinated accrediting activities formerly carried out by the National Organization for Public Health Nursing, the National League of Nursing Education, the Association of Collegiate Schools of Nursing, and the Council on Nursing Education of the Catholic Hospital Association.[59] The National Accrediting Service was responsible to the Joint Committee on Unification of Accrediting Activities, which included about thirty members representing the nursing organizations, the American Medical Association, the American Hospital Association, and the regional associations of higher education.[60] The Joint Committee, in turn, was responsible to the joint board of directors of the six national nursing organizations.[61]

For this second study of American schools of nursing, the National

Nursing Accrediting Service collected questionnaire data and conducted site visits. It also collected data from state boards of nursing, although this was voluntary.[62] Of the 904 basic programs that applied, 624 were approved for temporary accreditation for a period of five years and 276 were not approved.[63] The approved programs included 577 diploma and 51 degree programs. The list of temporarily accredited programs, which was subsequently published in the August 1952 issue of the *American Journal of Nursing,* resulted in an "eruption that . . . left few people in doubt about what it could mean not to appear on a list."[64]

A program of temporary accreditation continued until 1962, so that the majority of schools on the list could achieve full accreditation. Self-evaluation guides and regional conferences on topics related to curriculum, teaching, student selection, and welfare were sponsored by the Division of Nursing Education of the NLN, which assumed responsibility in 1952 for all nursing education accreditation activities in the United States.[65] Throughout the nine years during which the program of temporary accreditation continued, a program of full accreditation for all types of nursing programs, graduate as well as undergraduate, was carried on.[66] In 1952, the NLN Division of Nursing Education had two major departments: the Department of Baccalaureate and Higher Degree Programs and the Department of Diploma and Associate Degree Programs. Later on, a separate Department of Associate Degree Programs was established, as well as a Department of Practical Nurse Education.[67]

The success of nursing program accreditation in the United States is attested to partially by the increasing number and proportion of schools that achieved accreditation. A revised list of accredited programs published in the February 1950 issue of the *American Journal of Nursing* included 24 postgraduate, 34 public health, 35 collegiate, 113 diploma, and 10 "affiliating" programs.[68] Taken together, the accredited collegiate and diploma programs represented 12.6 percent of the 1,170 programs then in existence.[69] By 1974, there were 225 accredited baccalaureate programs, 433 accredited diploma programs (representing 67.6 percent of all existing degree programs), and 207 accredited associate degree programs (representing 46 percent of all existing associate degree programs).[70] In 1994, the number and proportion of accredited nursing programs had risen to 128, or 99.9 percent, of all diploma programs; 578, or 67 percent of all associate degree programs; and 1,186, or 79 percent of all baccalaureate programs.[71] In addition, in 1993, 205, or 84 percent, of all master's programs in nursing were also accredited.[72]

In comparison, in 1994 only one-third of Canada's 33 baccalaureate programs and none of its 13 master's and 122 diploma nursing programs were accredited. Low rates of baccalaureate program accreditation may be due in part to the newness of the CAUSN's national voluntary accreditation program, which has been in operation for less than a decade and which can only handle an average of three to four reviews per year. Lack of available accreditation for either master's or diploma nursing education accounts for nonaccreditation of these programs. Why does nursing program accreditation have such a different history in Canada? What are the reasons for such a different history of nursing program accreditation in two countries that appear, at least on the surface, to have so many similarities in nursing education and practice? The remainder of this article will outline some reasons for the differences in Canadian and American nursing accreditation history.

Reasons for Differences in Canadian and American Nursing Accreditation History

The underlying reason for the different histories of nursing program accreditation in Canada and the United States is the intrinsic difference in the political and social systems of the two countries. These social and political differences naturally support alternative public policies. In this context, public policy is defined as a long series of related choices (including decisions not to act) made by government bodies and officials.[73] Relevant post–World War II public policies include philosophies of accreditation, public or philanthropic financing of postsecondary education and health services, nursing association support, and emphasis on student access to programming.

PHILOSOPHY OF ACCREDITATION

In his book *Accreditation — A Struggle over Standards in Higher Education*, William Seldon stated that it has generally been accepted in the United States that educational institutions and programs of study require some type of monitoring and that such monitoring can and should be provided by nongovernmental agencies.[74] Gothler emphasized the significance of this prevailing philosophy for American nursing program accreditation by noting that "[t]he accreditation process in nursing is modeled after the process used for many years in higher education through the regional ac-

crediting bodies."[75] In Canada, there has been, and continues to be, no such pervasive philosophy.

The perception of the need for accreditation in American higher education is attested to by the large number of bodies whose role it is to evaluate programs and institutions and to publish lists of those that meet certain predetermined criteria or standards. These bodies exist at the state, regional, and national levels. There is also a consortium of accreditation agencies, the Council of Post-Secondary Accreditation (COPA). There are no comparable accreditation bodies in Canada. Instead, the government coordinates postsecondary education through provincial ministries and councils. Most provinces have some type of quasi-governmental coordinating body for postsecondary institutions, including universities, regional and community colleges, and technical institutes. In all provinces, postsecondary institutions are funded directly by provincial governments, and most universities, colleges, and technical institutes are governed by public rather than private boards. There are few private postsecondary educational institutions in Canada. Student tuition accounts for less than 20 percent of the operating costs of universities, colleges, and technical institutions, and tuition fees are regulated by provincial governments intent on facilitating student access to programs. Lacking an entrepreneurial approach to higher education, and given the extent of governmental and quasi-governmental coordination, Canada has had no tradition of accreditation for higher education. Thus, there has been no systemwide support for either the philosophy or the process of nursing program accreditation.

PHILANTHROPIC FINANCING

Establishing and maintaining programs of accreditation is expensive. Much of the funding for early work on nursing program accreditation in the United States came from philanthropic organizations such as the Rockefeller Foundation, the Commonwealth Fund, and the National Foundation for Infantile Paralysis.[76] Without philanthropic funding, it is questionable whether American nursing program accreditation would have developed as quickly or as extensively. In the United States, as in Canada, nursing schools themselves have been reluctant to pay the costs associated with establishing and maintaining programs of accreditation.

In Canada, there is no tradition of philanthropy associated with nursing education. Before diploma nursing programs were moved into provincial systems of postsecondary education, sponsoring hospitals paid their costs from general hospital revenues, which, after the implementation of

universal hospital insurance, came from the provincial ministries of health. From the period just after the Second World War until recently, hospital schools of nursing were funded from the health care budgets of the provinces, and there was no money for expensive "add-ons" such as accreditation. In most provinces, once diploma programs were transferred from hospitals into community colleges, the prevailing skepticism of community college administrators regarding evaluation of educational programs by outside agencies precluded budgeting and administrative support for nursing program accreditation. A similar situation existed in the United States when administrators of junior and community colleges initially opposed accreditation of early associate degree nursing programs by outside agencies; however, the linking of federal funding to program accreditation eventually overcame this resistance.[77] No comparable linking of federal funds to accreditation has ever existed in Canada. Such linkage would likely have been interpreted by provincial governments as the federal government's constitutional intrusion into provincial affairs, since under the British North America Act, control over education, health, and welfare was vested in the provincial rather than the federal government.

PROFESSIONAL NURSING SUPPORT

Provincial professional nursing associations historically have been reluctant to promote nursing program accreditation in Canada, possibly because of their vested interest in controlling the process for approving schools of nursing. In seven of ten Canadian provinces, the approval of schools of nursing has been legislatively vested with the professional nursing associations. In the other three provinces, provincial professional nursing associations have input into the approval of schools of nursing through membership or representation in the relevant provincial body or agency. In this way, professional associations directly influence approval criteria, standards, and processes. With limited financial and personnel resources available to address both approval and accreditation, provincial professional nursing associations have been more interested in and have relied more heavily on approval mechanisms rather than accreditation to improve nursing education. The diploma nurse educators' and administrators' unsatisfactory experience with the CNA-sponsored accreditation trial project of the early 1950s likely served to reinforce provincial associations' skepticism about the usefulness of a national program of accreditation for nursing education.

Historically, Canada has had a limited number of nursing associations that might have promoted nursing program accreditation. For example,

Canada never had a national association of diploma nurse educators, which might have explored accreditation from the perspective of hospital, community college, and independent diploma schools. A national association of university nurse educators, CAUSN, was established in 1942. One of the CAUSN's original goals, to develop standards for university nursing education in Canada, was accomplished in 1986 when it adopted a national program of voluntary accreditation for baccalaureate nursing education only. As a national affiliation of provincial nursing associations, the CNA could recommend but not enforce standards for diploma education. Although the CNA tried for two decades after the publication of the 1950 *Report of the Pilot Project for the Evaluation of Schools of Nursing in Canada* to initiate a national program of nursing education accreditation, it was unsuccessful.

ACCESS, NOT STANDARDIZATION
Throughout the first half of the twentieth century, Canada's emphasis has been on growth and expansion, with limited concern for evaluation or standardization of institutions and services, as is accomplished through accreditation. Although historically some economic competition between regions and provinces has existed, the inherent Canadian political and social philosophy has been equalization of opportunity. This has resulted in a predisposition to equalization payments between provinces; coordination of health, welfare, and educational services within provinces; and collaboration rather than competition. One overriding concern has been equal access to educational and social programs. Access to postsecondary education, including nursing, has not been predicated on the student's ability to pay. Tuition has been controlled by provincial governments and kept relatively low. Nursing programs usually existed in sufficient numbers to meet the demands of both students and employers without promoting competition. Such a nonentrepreneurial educational environment did not lend itself to the ranking of programs, as is accomplished through accreditation.

Conclusion

In North America, nursing education and practice reflect the national social and political systems in which they are embedded. Differing social values and political practices, expressed as public policies, have given rise to alternative educational structures and control mechanisms. Thus, in the United

States, accreditation of nursing education programs has been a significant strategy for evaluating nursing education programs, while in Canada, a pervasive atmosphere of government coordination of postsecondary education has resulted in limited accreditation of nursing education.

The differences in nursing accreditation between Canada and the United States may become smaller as the North American Free Trade Agreement reduces distinctions in national, social, and political practices. During the summer of 1994, accreditation was the subject of a meeting of Canadian, American, and Mexican national nursing associations and of a trilateral conference involving twelve professions.[78] The CAUSN and American and Mexican associations responsible for accreditation are working on a joint paper to identify the similarities and differences between these countries. Accreditation programs are seen as one means of assessing and guaranteeing the quality of nursing education so that North American countries can recognize the educational qualification, licensure, and certification status of professionals crossing national boundaries.

SHARON L. RICHARDSON, PHD, RN
Associate Professor
Faculty of Nursing
University of Alberta
Edmonton, Alberta
Canada T6G2G3
Phone: (403) 492-6252

Acknowledgments

The research for this article was supported by an Operating Grant from the Central Research Fund of the University of Alberta and a Facilitation Grant and Postdoctoral Award from the Alberta Foundation for Nursing Research.

Notes

1. The purposes of accreditation are variously stated by nurse educators but usually entail improving nursing education through establishing criteria and standards against which programs are measured. For examples of the alternative ways of stating the purposes and definitions of nursing program accreditation, see Jannetta MacPhail, "Monitoring Standards in Nursing Education," in *Canadian Nursing: Issues and Perspectives,* 2nd ed. (St. Louis: Mosby Year Book, 1991), 285–86; Nancy

Diekelmann, David Allen, Christine Tanner, Hernan Vera, Ann Gothler, Linda Moody, and Moira Shannon, *The NLN Criteria for Appraisal of Baccalaureate Programs: A Critical Hermeneutic Analysis* (New York: National League for Nursing, 1989); and CAUSN, *Accreditation Program* (Ottawa: CAUSN, 1986), 10–20.

2. Sister Denise Lefebvre, "What Is Accreditation?" *The Canadian Nurse* 53, no. 1 (January 1957): 19. See also MacPhail, 285–86.

3. William Dunn, *Public Policy Analysis: An Introduction* (Englewood Cliffs, N.J.: Prentice-Hall, 1981), 46–47.

4. Harvey Agnew, *Canadian Hospitals 1920 to 1970: A Dramatic Half Century* (Toronto: University of Toronto Press, 1974), 116.

5. George Weir, *Survey of Nursing Education in Canada* (Toronto: University of Toronto Press, 1932), 525.

6. Agnew, 118–19.

7. Weir, 116.

8. James Gibbon and Mary Mathewson, *Three Centuries of Canadian Nursing* (Toronto: Macmillan, 1947), 162.

9. Blanche Duncanson, "The Development of Nursing Education at the Diploma Level," in *Nursing Education in a Changing Society* (Toronto: University of Toronto Press, 1970), 111.

10. Agnew, 119–20.

11. Tony Cashman, *Heritage of Service: The History of Nursing in Alberta* (Edmonton: Alberta Association of Registered Nurses, 1965), 208–10.

12. Helen Mussallem, "Professional Nurses' Associations," in *Canadian Nursing Faces the Future,* 2nd ed., ed. Alice Baumgart and Jenniece Larsen (St. Louis: Mosby Year Book, 1992), 499.

13. Agnew, 120.

14. Ibid., 120–22.

15. Ibid., 120.

16. CNA, *The Leaf and the Lamp* (Ottawa: CNA, 1968), 88.

17. This interpretation is based on *Minutes of Executive Committee Meetings, 1942 to 1948,* Board of Directors Collection, CNA Archives, ARC WY 1 Cal C75m, Ottawa, Ontario, which outline CNA activities and expenditures of the federal government grant.

18. Helen Mussallem, *Spotlight on Nursing Education: The Report of the Pilot Project for the Evaluation of Schools of Nursing in Canada* (Ottawa: CNA, 1960), 9–12.

19. *CNA and Accreditation: Chronologic Highlights to April 1974 Updated to 1978,* Board of Directors Collection, CNA Archives, ARC Wy 1 CA1 C74m.

20. Ibid., 2. See also Frances McQuarrie, "Accreditation — What's on the Record?" *The Canadian Nurse* 52, no. 6 (June 1956): 443.

21. A. R. Lord, *Report of the Evaluation of the Metropolitan School of Nursing, Windsor, Ontario* (Ottawa: CNA, 1952).

22. "Evaluation of Schools of Nursing," *The Canadian Nurse* 46, no. 2 (February 1950): 113.

23. Mussallem, *Spotlight,* 11.

24. Ibid., 3.

25. Ibid., 81.

26. See *CNA and Accreditation*, CNA Archives, ARC WY 1Ca1 C74f, box B, 2.21, for identification of the numerous standing and task committees of CNA that were associated with the accreditation issue and that struggled unsuccessfully from 1962 to 1982 to mount a national program of accreditation.

27. *Report of the Executive Director to the Canadian Nurses Association Board of Directors, 28–30 October 1981*, Reports of the Executive Director Collection, CNA Archives, ARC WY 1 CA1 C25.

28. *Minutes of the Meeting of the Canadian Nurses Association Executive Committee, 25–27 October 1981*, Executive Committee of the Board of Directors Collection, CNA Archives, ARC WY 1 CA1 C76m.

29. *Minutes — CAUSN Council Meeting, November 11–12, 1982*, CAUSN Collection, Queens University Archives, box 2, p. 6, Kingston, Ontario.

30. *Accreditation and Nursing Education in Canada: Report Prepared for CNA Board of Directors*, Reports of the Board of Directors Collection, CNA Archives, ARC WY 1 CA1 C74f, box B2.21.

31. Ibid., 8.

32. See A. R. Lord, *Report of the Evaluation of the Metropolitan School of Nursing, Windsor, Ontario* (Ottawa: CNA, 1952); and W. Stewart Wallace, *Report of the Experiment in Nursing Education of the Atkinson School of Nursing, Toronto Western Hospital, 1950–1955* (Toronto: Toronto Western Hospital, 1955).

33. Government of Canada, *Royal Commission on Health Services, Volume I* (Ottawa: Queen's Printer, 1964), 239.

34. Marguerite Letourneau, *Trends in Basic Diploma Nursing Programs within the Provincial Systems of Education in Canada, 1964–1974* (PhD diss., University of Ottawa, 1975).

35. Ibid.

36. Agnew, 124.

37. Ibid.

38. Statistics Canada, *Revised Registered Nurses Data Series* (Ottawa: Government of Canada, 1980).

39. Gibbon and Mathewson, 342.

40. Janet Kerr, "A Historical Approach to the Evolution of University Nursing Education in Canada (1919 to 1974)," in *Canadian Nursing: Issues and Perspectives*, 2nd ed. (St. Louis: Mosby Year Book, 1991), 255.

41. B. L. Tunis, *In Caps and Gowns* (Montreal: McGill University Press, 1966), 48.

42. Helen M. Carpenter, *A Divine Discontent: Edith Kathleen Russell, Reforming Educator* (Toronto: Faculty of Nursing, University of Toronto, 1982), 41–45.

43. This calculation is derived from student enrollment figures for hospital training schools and basic baccalaureate programs in 1962 reported by Helen K. Mussallem in the Royal Commission on Health Services' Report, *Nursing Education in Canada* (Ottawa: Queen's Printer, 1964), 14, 91.

44. Peggy Anne Field, Shirley Stinson, and Marie-France Thibaudeau, "Graduate Education in Nursing in Canada," in *Canadian Nursing Faces the Future*, 2nd ed. (St. Louis: Mosby Year Book, 1992), 426–27.

45. *Report and Recommendations of the Working Group on Accreditation: Revised 6 September 1973*, CAUSN Collection 5073, Queens University Archives, box 5.

46. *Minutes of the Canadian Association of University Schools of Nursing Council Meeting, October 30–31, 1972*, CAUSN Collection 5073, Queens University Archives, box 2.

47. Ibid., 12.

48. *Minutes of the CAUSN Council Meeting, October 15 & 16, 1978*, CAUSN Collection 5073, Queens University Archives, box 2.

49. *Minutes of the CAUSN Council Meeting, November 24–25, 1981*, CAUSN Collection 5073, Queens University Archives, box 2.

50. Rondalyn Kirkwood and Jeannette Bouchard, *"Take Counsel with One Another": A Beginning History of the Canadian Association of University Schools of Nursing, 1942–1992* (Ottawa: CAUSN, 1992), 55.

51. J. E. F. Hastings, "Federal-Provincial Insurance for Hospital and Physician's Care in Canada," in *Perspectives on Canadian Health and Social Services Policy: History and Emerging Trends* (Ann Arbor: Health Administration Press, 1980), 198–219.

52. Helen Nahm, "What We Have Learned in the United States from More Than Thirty Years of Accreditation of Nursing Schools," speech to CAUSN, June 1974, CAUSN Collection 5073, Queens University Archives, box 5.

53. Ibid., 3.

54. Ibid.

55. Ibid., 4.

56. "Interim Classification of Schools of Nursing," *American Journal of Nursing* 49 (October 1949).

57. Nahm, 4.

58. Ibid., 1

59. Ibid.

60. Ibid., 1–2.

61. Ibid., 2.

62. Ibid., 5–6.

63. Ibid., 6.

64. Ibid.

65. Ibid., 2.

66. Ibid., 7.

67. Ibid., 2.

68. "Accredited Programs in Nursing," *American Journal of Nursing*, 50 (February 1950).

69. Nahm, 5.

70. Ibid., 12.

71. NLN, *Nursing Data Source, Volume 1, 1994* (New York: NLN, 1994).

72. NLN, *Nursing Data Source, Volume 2, 1993* (New York: NLN, 1993).

73. Dunn, 47.

74. William K. Seldon, *Accreditation — A Struggle over Standards in Higher Education* (New York: Harper Brothers, 1960).

75. Ann Gothler, "Accreditation — Past, Present, and Future," in *The NLN*

Criteria for Appraisal of Baccalaureate Programs: A Critical Hermeneutic Analysis, ed. Linda Moody and Moira Shannon (New York: NLN, 1989), 48.

76. Nahm, 5.

77. Ibid., 14.

78. Wendy McBride, "Executive Director's Message," *Canadian Association of University Schools of Nursing Newsletter* (Summer 1994): 3.

"We Are Left So Much Alone to Work Out Our Own Problems"

Nurses on American Indian Reservations During the 1930s

EMILY K. ABEL
School of Public Health
University of California, Los Angeles

Despite the recent flowering of public health history, federal American Indian health policy has received little attention. As Richard A. Meckel writes, "[I]f there is a monograph in desperate need of being written, it is one that will describe and analyze federal public health activity on Indian reservations."[1] Nurses hired by the Bureau of Indian Affairs (BIA) provide a good place to begin, because they were responsible for dispensing the great bulk of government health services to American Indians on reservations. This essay discusses these nurses and their work during the 1930s, focusing on their goals, the obstacles they encountered, and the accommodations they made.

The BIA nursing service grew rapidly during the 1930s, from 196 in 1929 to 596 in 1939. Approximately one-fourth of those in the service were public health nurses, dubbed "field nurses" to differentiate them from nurses employed by the Public Health Service.[2] In 1922, the BIA commissioned the American Red Cross to investigate the need for public health nurses on reservations. The report found extremely high morbidity and mortality rates and concluded that public health nurses could "assist in improving health conditions."[3] Two years later, the first three field nurses were hired.[4] The Merriam Report, conducted at the request of the secretary of the interior in 1928, recommended an enormous expansion of the field nursing service, arguing that "properly trained [nurses] could accomplish marvelous results [in] creating health habits for the prevention of illness and in raising living standards."[5]

Nevertheless, the staff initially grew slowly. Lack of funds prevented the BIA from offering salaries that were competitive with those in other

Nursing History Review 4 (1996): 43–64. Copyright © 1996 by The American Association for the History of Nursing.

government agencies and private practice.[6] Poor working conditions also deterred qualified women from applying. The nurses had large caseloads, were isolated from colleagues, had few resources at their disposal, lived in accommodations they considered substandard, and lacked opportunities for advancement. As one field nurse later commented, "BIA Nursing was the step child of all Gov't Services."[7] The BIA was able to fill all openings only during the Depression, when other positions were scarce.[8]

Some state and private agencies, such as the New Mexico Association on Indian Affairs and the Eastern Association on Indian Affairs, also provided funding for public health nurses.[9] Because the reports of such nurses are located with those of nurses hired by the BIA, I discuss them together. After examining the work of the field nurses, I briefly describe the work of nurses based in reservation hospitals and sanatoria.

Field Nurses

GOALS

Like other public health nurses, the field nurses were expected to downplay bedside nursing. A circular issued by the BIA in 1928 acknowledged that "some bedside care offers the greatest opportunity for getting the sympathy and understanding of the people." Nevertheless, the circular stressed that it would be "both impossible and unwise to make bedside care the greatest factor, as the hospitals should be used to a larger extent than is customary at present." One task of the field nurses was to "be a great influence in stimulating the use of the hospital." Other obligations of the field nurses included screening for such conditions as trachoma, tuberculosis, and sexually transmitted diseases, and providing immunizations. Above all, the BIA insisted that education was the field nurses' primary focus.[10]

By imparting information about disease causation, the nurses helped to democratize medical knowledge. Some components of health education, however, also furthered the goal of assimilation, providing avenues for inculcating Euro-American attitudes and values. "Diet, cleanliness, and ventilation are three big factors in the health condition here," wrote Alice J. Nelson, a nurse in Montana. "We are trying very hard to teach these things in the homes, classes and women's meetings." To promote cleanliness, the nurses encouraged American Indians not only to boil contaminated water before cooking with it, but also to landscape their yards and decorate the interior of their homes with wallpaper. Under the rubric of diet, the nurses taught how to plant household gardens, can fruits and vegetables, and cook

in the Euro-American style. When instructing new mothers, the nurses provided information about the intestinal and respiratory diseases that caused a high proportion of infant deaths. In addition, the nurses advised women to give babies English names, feed them by the clock, and make them sleep alone.[11]

Assuming a close relationship between personal habits and disease, the nurses were able to extend their purview as health educators still farther. Some focused on what they considered the high rate of out-of-wedlock births. "If there is anything more prominent than another in my ambition for our people," wrote LaDora White about the Apache in Oklahoma, "it is an earnest desire to create higher standards of living—getting our unmarried mothers married, giving a heritage of a father's love and care to the children, a more stable home and mother." Grace Olsen taught a Shawnee school girl "that she must be polite and obedient and considerate of others at all times if she expected to get along."[12]

If one goal of the nurses was to convince the Indians to accept Western medical care, another was to discourage them from demanding two types of services. A common complaint was that the Indians had "preconceived ideas" about the nurses' responsibilities, expecting them to be "pill peddlers" and "taxi drivers." Mollie Reebel, a nurse in Nava, New Mexico, wrote, "If I were given about fifty gallons each of Liniment and Cough Syrup, and an unlimited supply of Vaseline, would do a 'Land Office Business,' but following the policy outlined by the Office, have discouraged these." The nurses gave several reasons for refusing to fulfill medication requests; clients often administered medicine inappropriately, large supplies of drugs enabled them to bypass the nurses' authority, some medications could be prescribed only by physicians, and the clients' preoccupation with drugs undermined the nurses' health promotion program. Margaret Mary Schorn, a nurse stationed at the Tulalip agency, wrote, "These Washington Indians are great believers in drugs, pills, and liquid medicines for all aches and pains. It takes persistent tireless efforts to teach them that food, rest and personal hygiene have a great deal to do with minor illnesses."[13] It is also possible that the nurses wanted to distinguish themselves from BIA physicians, whose practice frequently considered primarily of dispensing drugs.[14]

The nurses' language suggests that old notions of pauperism also influenced their stance. Like nineteenth-century social reformers who believed that strict control of charity was necessary to prevent the "demoralization" of the poor, the field nurses condemned the "demanding" attitude of the Indians and their "constant begging" and warned of the dangers of "indis-

criminate giving." The implication was that access to pills not only under-mined health, but also retarded progress toward independence and self-reliance.[15]

The nurses' attitude about driving clients to hospitals and sanitaria reflected similar concerns. We will see that most nurses readily acknowl-edged that the great majority of transportation requests were justified. But in a few cases, the nurses attributed deception to American Indians, claim-ing that they asked for rides to specific destinations for social rather than medical reasons.[16] And several nurses insisted that the American Indians should learn to take care of themselves in this arena as in all others. Florence McClintock explained her refusal to drive patients this way: "The sooner they learn they have some responsibility to themselves the better." Clara O. Herm, a nurse in Rosebud, South Dakota, noted that she could have boosted attendance at a health survey clinic "had we adopted the policy of going out to bring the Indians to the clinic. But the plan has been to help the Indians help themselves."[17]

OBSTACLES

Several factors prevented the field nurses from adhering to their goals as faithfully as intended. One was the paucity of resources devoted to Ameri-can Indian health care. Federal funding for Indian health services varied dramatically during the 1930s, falling from a high of $4 million in 1932 to $3 million in 1935, and then rising to over $5 million in 1939. Nevertheless, throughout the decade, expenditures were far from adequate to provide the services the nurses considered essential.[18]

The shortage of sanatoria and hospitals was an especially serious prob-lem, since the nurses were expected to institutionalize clients for childbirth and serious sickness. As a result of New Deal building programs, the num-ber of institutions serving American Indians increased during the 1930s; by 1940, there were seventy general hospitals, with a combined bed capacity of 3,053, and eleven sanatoria, containing 1,200 beds. But occupancy rates re-mained extremely high. In many instances, field nurses convinced clients to enroll in institutions only to discover that no vacancies existed.[19] Marie B. Morris complained, "To persuade a family that hospitalization is the proper procedure and then receive word that 'there is no space available' is really defeating our purpose." Moreover, institutions were often hundreds of miles away. Margaret Mary Schorn reported that the closest hospital was located 500 miles from the reservation in Nevada where she worked. "This is a very great distance to take a Patient," she commented. The poor quality

of the cars and roads coupled with bad weather conditions made many journeys slow and dangerous. Nurses often concluded that patients were too weak to withstand the ordeal.[20]

Other medical services were also sparse. "Our plans for immunization went astray and have had to be postponed until we can get the necessary vaccine," reported Gertrude F. Hosmer in Elko, Nevada. In the absence of "cooling facilities for carrying serums into the field," Edna M. Hardsaw suspended diphtheria immunization in Rosebud, South Dakota. Laura B. Smith, a Montana nurse, wrote, "I have been asking for a good many things in the way of supplies ever since I have been in Browning, but there always seems to be a reason why I dont [*sic*] get them. One of the things that I wanted very much is a Baby Scale." Grace W. McDaniel, a nurse among the Cherokee, wrote that her "pre-natal program . . . could be very thorough if only we had the equipment for the field work." Without access to dentists, the nurses could not obtain treatment for the oral health problems they detected in screens. Esther Nelson wrote, "Many have infected teeth and gums with the resultant aches and pains. . . . Last Fall we had a Dentist who examined the pupils in two schools and before he could do any work he was detailed elsewhere."[21]

Inability to fulfill promises of medical assistance sometimes eroded the trust that is basic to authority. A supervising nurse visiting Elizabeth W. Forster in Red Rock, New Mexico, observed that the failure of the local physician to keep scheduled clinic appointments "weakens Miss Forster's position with the Indians and makes them feel that all white medicine is thoroughly unreliable."[22] Lydia T. King described the problems caused by the scarcity of immunizations for Navaho people in Arizona. One man brought his family to King's office for inoculations. King wrote,

> Not having serum and no funds to buy, I tried to explain why he would have to wait. They were terribly disappointed, having driven eight miles in a wagon, and all prepared to undergo, what to them, is something of an ordeal. Hundreds of preschool children and adults in this territory are unprotected, and I have in the past talked to them at their homes and any group where we meet, of the advisability of such protection, and urging it. Now they want it, and I have to make excuses that do not even sound convincing to myself.[23]

The shortage of some resources not only hindered the nurses' work, but also deprived them of the visible symbols of professional status. Arriving in Rocky Boy, Montana, Ruth Riss Seawright was "surprised to learn that . . . there was nothing to work with. I had no nursing bag. So I carried a galvanized bucket and a jug of soapy water." Many nurses held clinics in

partitioned rooms in their own living quarters. When examining children in Arizona, Lydia King was "obliged to use a corner of the school room."[24]

Patients' homes were the most common site for the delivery of care. Here nurses frequently confronted an extensive array of relatives, friends, and neighbors. Summoned to attend a delivery in New Mexico, Elizabeth Forster "found the hogan filled with an audience of men, women, and children." On another occasion she counted eighteen observers.[25]

According to Orpha Zoa Hall, a nurse in Pine Ridge, South Dakota, the presence of such a crowd "gives a splendid opportunity to demonstrate hygienic care and treatments of disease." But many members of the patients' entourage refused to acknowledge the nurses' claims to special expertise. Denied permission to bring a child with a nasal hemorrhage to the hospital, M. Gertrude Sturges packed the nose herself. Returning to the home a few hours later, she found that "they had removed the packing." Although Sturgis repacked the nose and applied ice, she could not convince the family of the merits of her treatment. At sundown, "the medicine man arrived and we were forced to give up and go away. Their comment was, 'the nurse was no good, nose packing was no good, I should have been able to give medicine to have stopped the bleeding.'" A recurrent complaint in the reports was that old people challenged the nurses' authority. Mollie Reebel reported that she was "most decidedly frosted" by a grandmother "who informed me through my interpreter that she knew as much about sickness and how to take care of it as any 'Bellacano' — American — and I might as well go home." Not surprisingly, some nurses sought to expel the neighbors and friends who flocked to medical events.[26]

Traditional healers could be even more intimidating. Arriving at the home of a birthing woman, Alice Clayton found the "situation somewhat complicated." According to Clayton, "the midwife was upset by my arrival, jealous of her dignity, and the fee she expected to get and I think she was afraid I would endanger both. I was quite determined to stay." Although a husband invited Seba Ates to attend a delivery, she realized she "was not received with much favor as the medicine man was there." Anna C. Phillips reported a similar encounter: "I noticed I was going to have some competition as there were two old Indian women present and they were ready to deliver the patient."[27]

In some cases, the nurses' lack of confidence in their own skills may have intensified their discomfort. The field nurses routinely complained that they were entrusted with responsibilities exceeding their competence. "We are left so much alone to work out our own problems," wrote Laura

Smith. Dorothy Loope later remembered her sense of unease when assuming her post at Fort Thompson, South Dakota: "I had worked in Texas as an institutional nurse and in Ann Arbor Michigan at the University Hospital and had taken some Public Health courses while there but did not have my certificate nor a degree. So I felt quite inadequate in this different work but I thought that surely there would be someone there who would advise me. But I soon learned that there wasn't."[28] Unlike urban public health nurses, the field nurses had no opportunities for regular contact with colleagues. Visits from supervisors were rare. Ruth Riss Seawright recalled, "I did not meet a supervising nurse until I had been in the service nearly two years."[29]

Contact with physicians was also limited. Even when full-time BIA physicians were stationed nearby, they rarely accompanied the nurses on home visits. Many nurses were dependent on the services of local doctors whom the government hired to work part-time on reservations; the willingness of these "contract doctors" to fulfill their obligations to American Indians varied enormously.[30] "Perhaps it is due to the fact that I am in such an out of the way place that Dr. Stevens has never visited my office or me in the field," wrote Alice D. Divine, a nurse for the Cheyenne and Arapaho Agency. "I can't help feeling that I would have been more successful in the things I was trying to accomplish if I had been able to freely talk over my problems with someone who was interested in them."[31]

Although trained to work under doctors' supervision, field nurses often found themselves alone making diagnoses, dispensing medicines, deciding on institutional placement, and managing births. When Ruth Riss Seawright began work, she asked the superintendent of her jurisdiction who dispensed medicines when the physician was away. He replied, "You do and God help you [if] you don't know what you are doing." Seawright later commented, "There I was 35 miles from the contract doctor and I had never given a patient 5 grains of aspirin without a doctors [*sic*] orders." Emergencies also tested Seawright's competence:

> One morning a small child was brought to clinic. The child was crying and had a bloody secretion around nose and mouth. The policeman . . . explained the child had inserted something into his nose and the mother had pushed it further in trying to remove it. I had never been asked to remove a foreign object from the nose. What could I do? I quickly prayed.[32]

Elizabeth Forster approached a delivery with trepidation. When the wife of her interpreter went into premature labor, Forster hurried to the house

to find that it was too late to think of taking Lilly thirty miles to the hospital for her delivery, as I had meant to do. I had to face the prospect of delivering her alone under what seemed most unfortunate conditions. I set about getting a fire made, water boiling and other necessary preparations, watching Lilly meanwhile. Difficulties threatened and I was relieved when the Trader sent word that he had his car out and was ready to start for the doctor at a word from me. I gave the word and he was off. In spite of haste, however, it was several hours before he could get back . . . , so that Lilly and I managed alone.[33]

The presence of doctors did not automatically restore confidence. According to the Merriam Report of 1928, the training of field nurses often was "considerably in advance" of that of the physicians employed by the BIA.[34] Moreover, many of the cases physicians attended required equipment and supplies that were unavailable in American Indian homes. "I must admit that my courage quailed when I contemplated the prospect of an instrumental delivery in a Navaho hogan," wrote Elizabeth Forster about her trip with both a doctor and interpreter to attend a woman who had been in labor for five days. "Throughout the trip I hoped desperately against hope that we might find the baby safely arrived or that we might be able to take the woman to the hospital." As Forster explained, "Navaho hogans are devoid of furniture of any description." Although she "managed to secure from a neighboring hogan two wooden fruit boxes which we utilized as operating table," this "elevated our patient only about six to eight inches, so it was necessary to work squatting on the dirt floor." Because Forster was the only medical assistant, she was responsible for administering anesthesia, a task normally considered inappropriate for nurses. The only light came from a fire, but this had to be extinguished before Forster could begin.

> We were therefore left without light, except that supplied by my small two-battery flash, which [the interpreter] operated, directing the light first to me as I administered ether, then to the doctor busy with his instruments. Back and forth, back and forth he darted the tiny light as we cried our need, and I prayed for a steady hand between flashes. Imagine our surprise and delight when we heard the lusty cry of a living and evidently husky baby.[35]

Other nurses helped doctors set limbs and perform surgery in equally difficult conditions. Surrounded by a variety of both formal and informal Indian practitioners, unsure of their own skills, and working in unfamiliar environments, many nurses were reluctant to be assertive.

Another factor weakening the status of the nurses was their dependence on client participation. The nurses generally initiated action in response to health problems that were brought to their attention, but some Indians sought to render illnesses and births invisible. One mother took aggressive steps to avoid detection. Seeing a nurse arrive, she "threw a blanket over the child." When the nurse "rashly . . . picked up the edge of the blanket to look under," the mother snatched it away and threatened the nurse with a knife. The day after Nettie Johnston Story attended a home birth, she learned that a family living in a back room of the house had remained hidden because their baby was gravely ill with pneumonia. Other parents reassured nurses that children were "all right," "fine," or "getting better" when death was imminent.[36]

Adults also concealed their own conditions. After noting that she brought a baby to the hospital, Anna May Swanson wrote, "The childs [*sic*] mother looked very thin to me in the firelight but she claimed that she was well. The following Sunday she passed away so she did not want me to know that she was ill at the time she sent her baby to the hospital for care." Despite the nurses' attempts at surveillance, many women successfully hid pregnancies and failed to notify the nurses when labor began. Screening programs occasionally enabled the nurses to circumvent the problem of relying on client reports, but obtaining consents for tests constituted still another hurdle. Patients and families also frequently disputed diagnoses.[37]

The greatest resistance was to institutionalization. Many American Indians who accepted the ministrations of nurses at home or in clinics rejected recommendations for placement in hospitals or sanatoria. "It is somewhat like trying to raise the dead," wrote Gertrude Hosmer about her attempts to persuade two tuberculous patients to enter a sanatorium in Nevada. Mollie Reebel voiced her frustration this way: "We travelled fifteen miles over the prairie, across a very rocky mesa where there was not even a wagon road. We found the patient, who was indeed very sick with symptoms indicating an acute abdominal condition, who after all our trip and over an hour trying to persuade him to go to the hospital which was his only hope, stubbornly refused."[38] The strongest opposition came from parents of young children. Report after report described confrontations with parents who refused to part with their offspring. "In some ways, this has been a very difficult month, perhaps the most of any I have experienced so far," wrote Ruth I. Peffley, explaining that a one-year-old child had developed bronchial pneumonia.

It was diagnosed at the very onset by the government doctor and urged to go to hospital. The family refused and three days later drove the babe fifty miles to an off the reservation doctor only to receive the same advice. . . . Finally after much manoeuvering and running about by the family, they were again approached concerning the hospital with the same negative reply. At the end of eight days the babe died. A deliberate sacrifice to false beliefs.[39]

Some clients avoided direct confrontations by verbally agreeing to enroll in institutions but failing to show up. H. Louisa Harple reported that a young woman twice promised to enter a sanatorium but never made preparations to go. Another common complaint was that American Indians postponed admission so long that they rendered treatment ineffective. Instead of going to the hospital at the first sign of labor, birthing women waited until they encountered serious difficulties. Tuberculous patients refused even to consider entering sanatoria until their diseases were advanced. And parents kept sick children at home until the optimal time for correcting their problems had passed. "Cases like this make one feel so sad," commented Anna May Swanson about a baby who died en route to the hospital. "The life of the baby could probably have been saved if the child had been brought in sooner or the physician or nurse notified but they usually wait until there is no hope at home before they will accept medical help."[40]

To be sure, many American Indians embraced the services the nurses offered. "I am thrilled about the pre-natal work," wrote Clara Cunningham. "I have brought 5 patients in to the hospital this month for pre-natal examinations. 3 of them not more than 6 months pregnant." According to Margaret Mary Schorn, "The Acoma Indians love to go to the hospital, are gracious when confined, thankful when they leave, and anxious to return." Alice D. Divine observed the fruits of her health education work: "I was amazed at some of the places I visited. Doors and windows had recently been screened, the yards cleaned and free from rubbish."[41]

But acceptance was rarely secured once and for all. Some families built screens but continually propped them open. Women who consented to attend prenatal classes frequently refused to prepare for the baby or called midwives for the birth. And many people who began treatments for such conditions as trachoma or sexually transmitted diseases discontinued them early.[42]

Resistance also continued after institutionalization. Sara Marie F. Babb reported an "exultant thrill of pride" after persuading a patient suffering from pneumonia to go to the hospital. "But my triumph was brief," she wrote. "After three days the patient deserted the hospital in disgust, declar-

ing Indian medicine was better." Retention was an equally serious problem in sanatoria. Margaret Mary Schorn wrote, "A very trying situation confronts us in that the parents of tubercular children take the patients out of the sanatorium against advice. The little tots go back into the contaminative, unhygienic homes and peculiar habits, some descript and some nondescript and the splendid work of the sanatoria is completely obliterated."[43]

Even a long institutional stay did not necessarily mean that American Indians had converted to Western medicine. Nor could successful outcomes guarantee that a nurse's victory was unambiguous. "On one home visit," Anna May Swanson reported, "found a small child with a kidney complaint but the parents refused to have doctor called or take child to hospital although less than a year ago the sight on this same child was saved in the hospital." Swanson commented, "When one finds cases of this sort and are [sic] unable to do anything to help it makes you wonder if you are really accomplishing anything when you work so hard to try to help."[44]

In a few extreme cases, nurses mobilized state power to force compliance. Most coercive measures were directed at parents. One parent who refused to obtain medical care for a child was threatened with loss of relief, another with denial of custody, and a third with charges of neglect. But instances of compulsion were rare. According to the medical director of the BIA in 1929, nurses and doctors were expected to practice "persuasive measures" rather than "coercive efforts."[45]

Unable to exert authority over their clients, many nurses trod warily. One supervisor applauded a nurse who responded "very cautiously" to her clients' requests. Laura Smith described her "fear and trembling" when asking a grandmother's permission to hospitalize a child with a high fever. Elizabeth Forster refrained from suggesting surgery to a patient until she felt that she was "sufficiently well established in [his] good graces." Others also paid close attention to the cues emanating from their clients, carefully noting which actions enhanced their "popularity" and which fostered "unfriendliness" or "antagonism." As Arvila Manthey wrote, "The Health Conservation Program is entirely dependent upon the good will of a people."[46]

PRACTICES

Constrained both by the attitudes of their clients and the lack of resources, many nurses adjusted their strategies. After reporting her failure to convince two Shawnee parents in Oklahoma to send their sick child to a hospital, Anna C. Holliday commented, "In that case we just have to do the best

we can." Esther Nelson wrote in a similar vein when she found all Navaho hospitals full during a measles epidemic: "Under the circumstances we did the best we could." Although the nurses could ignore the limitations imposed by the context when articulating their goals, they stressed the need for flexibility when reporting their activities.[47]

Doing "the best" that was possible often meant providing bedside nursing. Although the BIA had hoped that institutionalization would render much of that care unnecessary, virtually all nurses spent many hours ministering to sick patients at home. When Ida E. Rix was unable to take a sick Choctaw baby in Mississippi to the hospital, she "wrapped the baby well in blankets and placed warm irons around him" and in general "gave all the care possible in the home." Gertrude Hosmer described her experience with an elderly Oklahoma woman: "The family would not consider hospitalization because they wanted her to leave from her own home. Giving her care in her own home was truly difficult and required from one to two hours daily towards the last." As we have seen, many nurses attended home births, despite their commitment to hospital deliveries. The barriers to institutionalization also compelled some nurses to violate their own injunctions against dispensing medicine. For example, Edna P. Holzworth, an Arizona nurse, wrote that she found "one baby, quite sick, but mother refused Hospt. nurse gave cough med. Milk mag. and oint. to apply to chest."[48]

In addition, most nurses broke their rules about driving. Very few Indians had cars. As already noted, the closest hospitals and sanatoria often were hundreds of miles away. And a high proportion of Indians lived too far to be able to walk to outpatient facilities. Virtually all nurses thus devoted much of their work week to transporting clients to medical services.

The demands of home nursing care and transportation often left little time for health education. "I find discouragement in the fact that I am doing no constructive education work," wrote Cecilia Severino, "that I am too busy doing first aid, emergency work and sick calls." Most nurses attempted to integrate health education and care of the sick, but they rapidly realized that their work could not have the exclusively educational focus the BIA deemed essential.[49]

Nurses jettisoned their original precepts most radically by making accommodations to traditional healing practices. The BIA was committed to substituting White medicine for Indian healing practices. Nevertheless, some nurses facilitated the work of Indian healers by giving them advice

and supplies. Louise O. Kuhrtz, a New Mexico nurse, reported, "The head mid-wife of the village comes to me for supplies, argyrsol, bandage, and rubbing alcohol. She cooperates very well and has a good degree of success. This past year not a single mother was lost." Josephine L. Shefner, a nurse in Rosebud, South Dakota, provided a midwife with scissors to improve her method of severing the umbilical cord. Nurses occasionally acknowledged that the knowledge transfer went both ways. Describing a midwife she had known well during her early years as a field nurse, Ruth Riss Seawright commented, "I learned from her and she learned from me."[50]

Some nurses delivered care alongside traditional healers. Elizabeth Forster wrote that when an old Indian man was ill, she made several trips to "consult and collaborate with the Medicine Man who has been singing for him." Forster expressed unusual respect for American Indian healers in letters to friends and relatives; her willingness to ally herself with the "Medicine Man" is thus perhaps unsurprising. But even nurses who did not share Forster's appreciation for traditional practitioners occasionally worked with them. M. Jane West, a Montana nurse, explained why she agreed to a healer's request that she attend his daughter's confinement. "The delivery was a hard one and needed both Dr. and nurse, as well as the Medicine Woman. I believe we will get farther with the Indians by adding to what is good in their religious practices than by ignoring the Medicine Man and Woman entirely." After describing a woman who was convinced she had been "witched," Mollie Reebel wrote, "My 'compadre' the 'Witch Doctor' and I work side by side for several hours, trying to talk her out of this idea." Reebel also solicited the assistance of a "medicine man" in the case. When Charlotte Conrad brought a distraught young mother and her dying baby home from the hospital, Conrad "did the only human thing left to do — I brought their medicine man to them." Still another nurse provided aid while waiting for an American Indian practitioner to arrive. Esther Nelson cared for a woman struck by lightning until the traditional ceremony began the following morning.[51]

Arriving at homes in the midst of "sings," some nurses fled in horror; others, however, waited for the ceremonies to end, and a few administered aid or arranged hospital care while traditional rituals were in progress. "An interesting experience happened one evening this week," wrote Dorothy J. Williams. Asked to visit a Navaho hogan, she found a dying woman and immediately began providing care. "All the time I was working with her, the medicine men were singing and making motions toward her with their

hands," Williams noted. If isolation occasionally undermined the nurses' confidence, it also gave them freedom to work out their own relationships with the indigenous healers they encountered.[52]

Home births provided particularly important lessons in negotiation. The nurses had to listen to the various voices in the room and modify their actions accordingly. One nurse who encountered two midwives already present at a birth claimed that she "ignored their method of delivery."[53] But disregarding Indian practices was rarely an option. Summoned to help a midwife deliver a baby, Elizabeth Forster "had mostly to do the lady's bidding," although she was "able to introduce a few hygienic measures of my own."[54]

In many cases, the nurses' participation was restricted to the postpartum period. Mattie C. Haywood recoiled from the practices she saw in New Mexico. "It's astonishing that mother or babe ever survive," she wrote. "Modern zoological methods transcend their procedure." Nevertheless, she could be "scarcely more than a witness." After the birth, however, she was able to provide some care for the infant. More commonly, the nurses were excluded from the births but called in afterward to deliver specific types of care, such as extracting the placenta, applying silver nitrate to the baby's eyes, and dressing the cord.[55]

Although the nurses tended to be more welcome after the baby had been born than before, few enjoyed undisputed authority at any time. A major goal of the field nurses was to encourage women to lie prone both during and immediately after birth. When Elizabeth Forster arrived at a home "just too late for the actual delivery," she found the birthing woman "held in a kneeling position by means of straps from the ceiling attached to each wrist." From Forster's perspective, the woman "looked none too comfortable"; nevertheless, Forster "was not allowed to release her for rest until after the birth of the placenta." Although Forster was "allowed to do the umbilical dressing and rub the wee one with oil," she had to heed the instructions of the "old woman who seemed mistress of ceremonies." Forster was "firmly bidden" to hold the baby over a "trough of sand prepared on the hogan floor while an attendant poured first cold then warm water over the little body, and the old lady rubbed it vigorously. . . . You may believe it or not," Forster concluded, "but the result was a fresh pink-tan baby who was then dressed in swaddling bands with arms pinioned to its sides, as all good Navaho babies are, and laid in its mother's arms."[56]

The nurses reported making other concessions as well. Although most

were determined to bathe newborn babies, several could not overcome the opposition of the birthing woman or her other attendants. Care of the umbilical cord constituted another source of contention. Eva Harting, a nurse in Montana, wrote, "One midwife left an umbilical cord 10 inches long attached to the infant, and when I suggested shortening it she and the mother both became quite agitated: 'The baby will get sick if you cut the cord any shorter.' I didn't shorten it." Harting explained her willingness to compromise: "If I had insisted, in all probability, this family would have refused me admission at my next call." Anna Phillips tied rather than shortened the cord of a Minnesota infant with a bleeding umbilicus in deference to the wishes of the mother who "was very much excited."[57]

There were limits to the ability of the nurses to accommodate traditional healing practices. Elizabeth Forster's willingness to work "hand in hand" with American Indian healers antagonized the BIA superintendent and was an important factor in her dismissal in 1933. Ignorance of American Indian practices also hindered cross-cultural exchange. The nurses typically arrived on reservations knowing little or nothing about the people they expected to serve. Although some sought opportunities to learn about indigenous cultures, others saw no reason to do so. Language differences contributed to the lack of understanding. All BIA schools taught English, but many older American Indians spoke only their own languages. Although most nurses were able to rely on patients' family or friends to translate, some acknowledged that communication through interpreters was extremely restricted. Only the rare nurse sought to learn an American Indian language. Nevertheless, circumstances compelled the nurses to attend to the wishes of their clients as much as possible.[58]

Institutional Nurses

We might expect nurses in hospitals and sanatoria to have had greater success in imposing their authority. They delivered care on their own turf and had regular contact with other White practitioners. Interviews conducted with former institutional nurses in the 1970s demonstrate, however, that they encountered many of the problems that beset field nurses and responded in similar ways.

The low level of federal funding for Indian health services meant that all BIA institutions had serious deficiencies. According to the 1935 Annual

Report of the Phoenix Sanatorium, "The crying need of the entire institution . . . is an increase in the operating allotment. For the past fiscal year the per diem cost per patient was less than $1.50."[59] Ethyle Denton, a nurse at the Phoenix Indian Hospital during the 1930s, later wrote, "When I first saw the Indian Hospital I could hardly believe what I saw! . . . To say it was antiquated is putting it mild." Janet Green, a former hospital nurse at Fort Wingate, New Mexico, remembered the building as a "horror." The men's ward "had a vertical crack six or seven feet high and inches wide that we had to keep stuffed with newspapers."[60]

The sparse equipment tended to be grossly inadequate. Hospital nurses routinely used stoves for sterilization. Carrie Brilstra was astonished to discover that the sanatorium at Dulce, New Mexico, had four thermometers for eighty-eight patients and that the X-ray films were "unreadable."[61]

Understaffing was another problem. Most hospitals and sanatoria had only one doctor. If he quit unexpectedly or was temporarily absent, the nurses had to assume his responsibilities. Janet Green wrote, "One special case we had was an OB who came in with severe erysipelas and was delivered of twins. . . . Of course the doctor was away and I had to deliver them. I prayed hard that they would get no infection." Ruth Sperling treated a young Navaho sheepherder who arrived at a New Mexico hospital with a snake bite after the doctor had left for the weekend.[62]

Even when doctors were present, nurses were entrusted with responsibilities for which they considered themselves unprepared. Martha Keaton, a hospital nurse in Clinton, Oklahoma, in 1934, later gave this account: "One of the events I remember about my year . . . was that the doctor got an infected finger and a woman came in in labor. Instead of calling another doctor I as the nurse on duty had to deliver the baby. I was so mad and scared."[63] In hospitals, as in Indian homes, the responsibility for administering anesthesia also fell to nurses. "I believe, that at Jicarillo Apache Hospital, Dulce, N.M., I broke about every rule a nurse learned at Presbyterian Hospital in Chicago where I trained," wrote Ruth Burr.

> A most important one—A nurse is *not* to give anaesthetics. But in Dulce there was a doctor, a head nurse, and a night nurse—Me! An Employee's two children . . . needed Tonsillectomies so Dr. Howard Cornell told me I should pour ether while Cornelia R. McKam, R.N. would be his nurse. I had had a 12-hour shift of duty but got up from my sleep to "Pour Ether." I was scared, but he said he'd tell me to stop when patient had had enough, and showed me how to do it. So I poured. He got interested in his surgery so forgot me until his patient became a little blue. All surgery discontinued until breathing was restored. After that I learned the signs of anaesthesia.[64]

Returning to a Pennsylvania hospital for retraining, Ethyle Denton "shocked the nurses there" by describing the tasks she had been assigned at a BIA hospital.[65]

The shortage of ancillary staff created other difficulties. The nurses were frequently outraged to learn that they were expected to perform many chores they considered unbecoming to professionals. If the responsibility for delivering skilled medical services engendered insecurity, the need to stoke furnaces, wash dishes, and iron uniforms threatened to erode status differentials between nurses and patients. In short, the inadequacy of both material resources and personnel weakened the ability of the nurses to impose professional norms.

In addition, the nurses frequently encountered patient hostility. As we have seen, many American Indians enrolled in institutions reluctantly and left before the recommended discharge date. The nurses thus had an incentive to seek to win the patients' favor. In the hospital as at home, birthing women won important concessions. Some rejected delivery tables, retained kneeling positions, and even refused to accept the doctors' ministrations. In addition, some nurses allowed family members to remain with patients throughout their stays.[66] This in turn meant that hospital nurses, like their counterparts in the field, sometimes delivered care in the presence of onlookers. In addition, family members imposed extra burdens. "We had to bed them all down and feed them," Ruth Burr remembered.[67]

Hospital nurses also resembled field nurses in making accommodations to traditional healers. Although the nurses had hoped that institutional care would demonstrate the superior efficacy of White medicine, other practitioners were not excluded. Nealtha J. Stone recalled that a healer was given space in the hospital to conduct a special ceremony for two patients who had been struck by lightning. Darline Shewell appears to have turned a blind eye to healers who administered medicine to patients during visiting hours. "In order to encourage hospitalization," Ruth Burr explained, "we put up with their superstitions, taboos, etc."[68]

Conclusion

Nurses working on American Indian reservations during the 1930s faced overwhelming obstacles. They were expected not just to deliver health services but also to inculcate Euro-American patterns of thought and behavior. Most, however, lacked adequate resources and support. Many clients re-

tained critical distance from the nurses' authority, rejecting their educational advice and recommendations for institutionalization.

The nurses responded to structural constraints and client resistance by adapting their agenda. Field nurses dispensed medicine, drove clients to hospitals and sanatoria, and administered bedside care. Institutional nurses allowed relatives to stay with patients. Members of both groups accommodated traditional healers and accepted the durability of old forms in the face of the new.

It would be wrong to romanticize the nurses' interactions with their clients. The great majority remained ignorant about indigenous cultures and convinced of the superiority of Euro-American ways. BIA policies inhibited the rare nurse who expressed admiration for American Indian values and practices or sought to treat traditional healers as partners.

Nevertheless, the nurses' story points to a need to study the activities as well as the writings of individual health providers. It is much easier to locate manuals and other prescriptive literature than to uncover evidence of actual behavior. Moreover, the recent "linguistic turn" in scholarship has reinforced historians' preoccupation with rhetoric.[69] The experiences of nurses employed on American Indian reservations during the 1930s remind us that practice can diverge dramatically from rhetoric and is of equal, perhaps greater, importance. Nurses who expected American Indians to be passive consumers of Western knowledge and predefined services were compelled to acknowledge their agency. Although the nurses remained dominant, the clients often shaped the interactions. Unable to impose White medicine unilaterally, the nurses negotiated.

EMILY K. ABEL
Associate Professor
School of Public Health
University of California, Los Angeles
10833 Le Conte Avenue
Los Angeles, Calif. 90024-1772
Phone: (310) 395-0674

Acknowledgments

This article was funded by the UCLA Center for the Study of Women and the UCLA Center for American Indian Studies. I wish to thank Leigh Pruneau for generously sharing her own research on field nurses, and Richard L. Abel, Carole H. Browner, Joan E. Lynaugh, and Nancy Reifel for reading and commenting on an earlier draft.

Notes

1. Richard A. Meckel, "Judging Progressive-Era Infant Welfare in Light of *Fatal Years* — and Vice Versa," *Bulletin of the History of Medicine* 68, no. 1 (Spring 1994): 110.

2. Ruth M. Raup, *The Indian Health Program from 1800 to 1955* (Washington, D.C.: U.S. Department of Health, Education, and Welfare, 1959), 12–13, 30.

3. Florence Patterson with Elizabeth Fox, *A Study of the Need for Public Health Nursing on Indian Reservations* (American Red Cross, 1924), 631.

4. Martha A. Sandweiss, ed., "Introduction," in *Denizens of the Desert, a Tale and Picture of Life Among the Navaho Indians: The Letters of Elizabeth W. Forster/ Photographs by Laura Gilpin* (Albuquerque: University of New Mexico Press, 1988), 18.

5. Brookings Institution, *The Problem of Indian Administration: Report of a Survey* (Baltimore: Johns Hopkins University Press, 1928), 24.

6. Brookings Institution, 189. See also Elinor D. Gregg, *The Indians and the Nurse* (Norman: University of Oklahoma Press, 1965), 89.

7. Ruth Riss Seawright to Virginia Brown and Ida Bahl, 20 January 1978, Brown, Ball and Watson Collection, Special Collections and Archives, Cline Library, Northern Arizona University, Flagstaff.

8. Raup, 10.

9. See Raup, 12–13; and Sandra Schackel, *Social Housekeepers: Women Shaping Public Policy in New Mexico, 1920–1940* (Albuquerque: University of New Mexico Press, 1992), 61–85. The field nurses sent both monthly and annual reports to Washington. These reports consisted of a two-page statistical section, in which the nurses enumerated the services they rendered, and a longer narrative section, in which they delineated their goals, chronicled their activities, and discussed individual cases. The reports are located in the records of the Bureau of Indian Affairs file E779, RG 75, National Archives. Individual reports are identified by the nurse's name, the name of the agency where she was stationed, and the date. A major source of information about both field nurses and institutional nurses is the collection of interviews conducted during the 1970s by Ida Bahl, a former BIA nurse. Bahl sent questionnaires to all nurses whose names she obtained in a "snow-ball" approach. Forty-eight women responded. Many not only answered the specific questions she posed, but also sent long letters describing their experiences. The original responses are now located in the Brown, Bahl, and Watson Collection.

10. Department of the Interior, "General Information on Nursing in the Indian Service (April 1928)," Brown, Ball, and Watson Collection. See Barbara Melosh, *"The Physician's Hand": Work Culture and Conflict in American Nursing* (Philadelphia: Temple University Press, 1982), 125.

11. Alice J. Nelson, "Monthly Report," Rocky Boy Agency, Mont., March 1934. Naomi Rogers notes that although early twentieth-century campaigns for cleanliness were couched in the language of scientific medicine, they were fraught with old assumptions about the relationship between dirt and disease. See *Dirt and Disease: Polio Before FDR* (New Brunswick, N.J.: Rutgers University Press, 1992).

12. LaDora White, "Monthly Report," Apache Agency, Okla., March 1935; Grace Olsen, "Monthly Report," Shawnee Agency, Cushing, Okla., Aug. 1934.

13. Mollie Reebel, "Monthly Report," Western Navaho Agency, Ariz., June 1936; Margaret Mary Schorn, "Monthly Report," Tulalip Agency, Wash., April 1933.

14. Brookings Institution, 234.

15. See Emily K. Abel, "Middle-Class Culture for the Urban Poor: The Educational Thought of Samuel Barnett," *Social Service Review* 52, no. 4 (December 1978): 596–620.

16. See, for example, Gregg, 101; and Cecilia Severino, "Monthly Report," Leupp Agency, Ariz., May 1935.

17. Florence McClintock, "Monthly Report," Sacramento, Calif., December 1934; Clara O. Herm, "Annual Report," Pine Ridge, S.D., 1933–1934.

18. Raup, 30.

19. See Gregg, 147; Raup, 30; and Esther F. Martin, "Monthly Report," Kiowa Agency, Okla., October 1935.

20. Marie B. Morris, "Monthly Report," Umatilla Agency, Pendleton, Oregon, September 1934; Margaret Mary Schorn, Carson, Nev., May 1934. See Stephen J. Kunitz, *Disease Change and the Role of Medicine: The Navajo Experience* (Berkeley: University of California Press, 1983), 147. The few community facilities located close to reservations rarely admitted Indians. See Raup, 9.

21. Gertrude F. Hosmer, "Monthly Report," Elko, Nev., May 1934; Edna M. Hardsaw, "Monthly Report," Rosebud, S.D., May 1934; Laura B. Smith, "Monthly Report," Browning, Mont., December 1934; Grace W. McDaniel, "Monthly Report," Cherokee, Okla., May 1934; Esther Nelson, "Annual Report," Eastern Navaho, Ariz., 1934–1935.

22. Quoted in Sandweiss, 12. Forster was employed by the New Mexico Association on Indian Affairs. For an account of her work, see Mary Ann Ruffing-Rahal, "The Navajo Experience of Elizabeth Forster, Public Health Nurse," *Nursing History Review* 3 (1995): 173–88.

23. Lydia T. King, "Monthly Report," Navaho Agency, Klagetoh, Ariz., December 1935.

24. Ruth Riss Seawright to Virginia Brown, 29 December 1980, Brown, Bahl, and Watson Collection; Lydia T. King, "Monthly Report," Southern Navaho, Arizona, 31 January 1934.

25. Elizabeth W. Forster to Laura Gilpin, 7 July 1932, in Sandweiss, 96; Elizabeth W. Forster, "Monthly Report," Shiprock, N.M., 7 November 1932.

26. Orpha Zoa Hall, "Monthly Report," Pine Ridge, S.D., October 1931; M. Gertrude Sturges, "Monthly Report," Say-nos-tee, June 1935; Mollie Reebel, Nava, N.M., December 1934. See Elizabeth W. Forster to Marion Gilmore, 18 February 1932, in Sandweiss, 68.

27. Alice Clayton, "Monthly Report," Ponca City, Okla., May 1934; Seba Ates, "Monthly Report," Leupp Agency, Ariz., July 1933; Anna C. Phillips, "Monthly Report," Cloquet, Minn., August 1932.

28. Laura B. Smith, "Monthly Report," Browning, Mont., July 1934; response of Dorothy Loope, "Questionnaire, Nursing Personnel Originals, Brown, Ball, and Watson Collection.

29. Response of Ruth Riss Seawright, "Questionnaire."

30. Raup, 12.

31. Alice D. Divine, "Monthly Report," Cheyenne and Arapaho Agency, Okla., February 1936.

32. Response of Ruth Riss Seawright, "Questionnaire."

33. Elizabeth Forster to Marion Gilmore, 30 December 1931, in Sandweiss, 59–60.

34. Brookings Institution, 249.

35. Elizabeth Forster to Marion Gilmore, 18 February 1932, 66–68.

36. Eva Harting, "Monthly Report," Tongue River Agency, Mont., August 1933; Nettie Johnston Story, "Monthly Report," Carson Agency, Nev., January 1932. According to John Duffy, immigrants in New York City who admitted nurses to their homes occasionally hid their sick. See *A History of Public Health in New York City, 1866–1966* (New York: Russell Sage, 1974), 263. On concealment as a form of resistance, see Michael Bloor and James McIntosh, "Surveillance and Concealment: A Comparison of Techniques of Client Resistance in Therapeutic Communities and Health Visiting," in *Readings in Medical Sociology,* ed. Sarah Cunningham-Burley and Neil P. McKeganey (London: Tavistock/Routledge, 1990), 159–81.

37. Anna May Swanson, "Monthly Report," Fort Apache Agency, Whiteriver, Ariz., June 1936.

38. Gertrude F. Hosmer, "Monthly Report," Elko, Nev., April 1934; Mollie Reebel, "Monthly Report," Nava, N.M., April 1933.

39. Ruth I. Peffley, "Monthly Report," Browning, Mont., April 1934.

40. H. Louisa Harple, "Monthly Report," Red Lake Agency, Minn., July 1931; Anna May Swanson, "Monthly Report," Fort Apache Agency, Whiteriver, Ariz., July 1935.

41. Clara Cunningham, "Monthly Report," Consolidated Ute Agency, Colo., October 1935; Margaret Mary Schorn, "Annual Report," Southern Pueblos Agency, N.M., December 1933–July 1934; Alice D. Divine, "Monthly Report," Cheyenne and Arapaho Agency, Okla., April, 1935.

42. See Arvilla Manthey, "Monthly Report," Keams Canyon Agency, June 1935.

43. Marie F. Babb, "Monthly Report," San Carlos Agency, Ariz., April 1933; Margaret Mary Schorn, "Monthly Report," Tulalip Agency, Wash., April 1933.

44. Anna May Swanson, "Monthly Report," Fort Apache Agency, Whiteriver, Ariz., January 1935.

45. D. M. Guthrie, "The Health of the American Indian," *Public Health Reports* 44, no. 16 (April 1929): 948.

46. Adelia L. Eggerstine, "Report," Minn., 12 January 1933; Laura B. Smith, "Monthly Report," Blackfeet Agency, Mont., April 1935; Elizabeth Forster to Helen Eyre, 3 January 1933, in Sandweiss, 123; Arvila Manthey, "Monthly Report," South Pueblos, N.M., March 1932.

47. Anna C. Holliday, "Monthly Report," Shawnee Agency, Okla., July 1931; Esther Nelson, "Monthly Report," Eastern Navaho Agency, N.M., July 1935. For examples of other public health nurses who responded flexibly to the conditions they found, see Melosh, 136–37; Molly Ladd-Taylor, *Mother-Work: Women, Child*

Welfare, and the State, 1890–1930 (Urbana and Chicago: University of Illinois Press, 1994), 176–79.

48. Ida E. Rix, "Monthly Report," Choctaw Agency, Miss., December 1935; Gertrude F. Hosmer, "Monthly Report," Kiowa Agency, Lawton, Okla., June 1936; Edna P. Holzworth, "Monthly Report," Western Navaho Agency, Ariz., February 1934.

49. Cecilia Severino, "Monthly Report," Leupp Agency, Ariz., July 1935.

50. Louise O. Kuhrtz, "Annual Report," Isleta, N.M., 1934; Josephine L. Shefner, "Monthly Report," Rosebud, S.D., November 1935; response of Seawright, "Questionnaire."

51. Elizabeth Forster to Helen Eyre, 3 January 1933, in Sandweiss 123; M. Jane West, "Monthly Report," Blackfeet, Montana, July 1935; Mollie Reebel, "Monthly Report," Nava, N.M., February 1936; Charlotte Conrad, "Monthly Report," Cheyenne and Arapaho Agency, Okla., September 30, 1932; Esther Nelson, "Monthly Report," Eastern Navaho Agency, N.M., August 1935.

52. Dorothy J. Williams, "Monthly Report," Northern Navaho Agency, N.M., November 1935.

53. Anna C. Phillips, "Monthly Report," Cloquet, Minn., December 1932.

54. Elizabeth Forster, "Monthly Report," Shiprock, N.M., November 1932.

55. Mattie C. Haywood, "Monthly Report," Jicarilla Agency, Dulce, N.M., 7 May 1936.

56. Elizabeth Forster to Laura Gilpin, 7 June 1932, in Sandweiss, 96.

57. Eva Harting, "Monthly Report," Tongue River Agency, Ashland, Mont., December 1933; Anna C. Phillips, "Monthly Report," Cloquet, Minn., August 1932.

58. See Brookings Institution, 223; Gregg, 89; "Questionnaire"; Schackel, 80.

59. "Annual Report of the Phoenix Indian Sanatorium," 1 July 1935, Records of the Bureau of Indian Affairs, RG 75, National Archives, Pacific Southwest Region, Laguna Niguel, California. Response of Ethyle Denton, "Questionnaire."

60. Response of Janet Green, "Questionnaire."

61. Response of Carrie Brilstra, "Questionnaire."

62. Response of Green, "Questionnaire"; response of Ruth Sperling, "Questionnaire."

63. Response of Martha Keaton, "Questionnaire."

64. Response of Burr, "Questionnaire."

65. Response of Denton, "Questionnaire."

66. Brookings Institution, 286.

67. Response of Burr, "Questionnaire."

68. Response of Stone, "Questionnaire"; response of Darline Shewell, "Questionnaire"; response of Burr, "Questionnaire."

69. See Kathleen Canning, "Feminist History After the Linguistic Turn: Historicizing Discourse and Experience," *Signs* 19, no. 2 (Winter 1994): 368–404.

Satisfied to Carry the Bag

Three Black Community Health Nurses' Contributions to Health Care Reform, 1900–1937

MARIE O. PITTS MOSLEY
Bellevue School of Nursing
Hunter College

Since the early twentieth century, community health agencies and visiting nursing organizations in New York City have employed a number of outstanding Black nurses. Among these exceptional women were three pioneers: Jessie Sleet, the first paid district Black nurse in New York City[1] and the first Black public health nurse in the United States[2]; Elizabeth Tyler, the first Black nurse hired as a visiting nurse by the Henry Street Settlement Visiting Nursing Service[3]; and Edith Carter, a senior nurse at Henry Street for twenty-eight years.[4]

This article shows that these three Black community health nurse pioneers made significant contributions to the development of New York City's community health nursing by providing much-needed health care to hundreds of unserved members of the Black community, providing strong leadership in their roles as supervisors, administrators, and educators in patients' homes, babies' health stations, settlement houses, and clinics.

A Successful Experiment: Jessie Sleet, First Black Public Health Nurse

In October 1900, Dr. Edward T. Devine, general secretary of the Charity Organization Society's (COS) tuberculosis committee, met with members of his committee to discuss the spiraling death rates from tuberculosis in the city and the high incidence of tuberculosis among the city's Black population. Prior to this, Dr. Devine had studied the health crisis among the city's Blacks and tried to come up with possible solutions to help eliminate the

Nursing History Review 4 (1996): 65–82. Copyright © 1996 by The American Association for the History of Nursing.

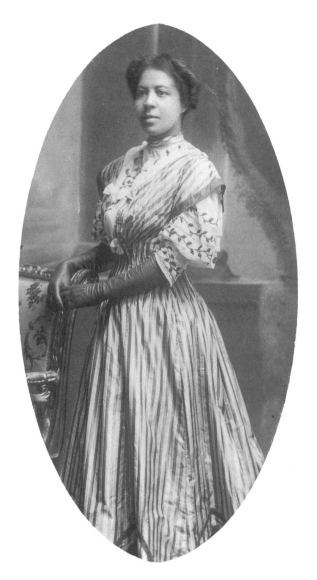

Figure 1. Jessie Sleet Scales. (By permission of Dr. M. Elizabeth Carnegie)

problem. Knowing that tuberculosis was a preventable disease born from lack of knowledge, he determined that in order to alleviate the poor health that seemed to be embedded in the Black community's life, a district nurse who was of the same race should be hired. This nurse would go into the Black communities both to do district visiting and to persuade the people to accept treatment.[5] Having never had any Black person in their organization, the COS's tuberculosis committee was disinclined to change their policies. Dr. Devine was finally able to convince the committee members of the benefits of having a Black nurse on the staff, but their consent came with a number of conditions. First, they would not be responsible for her salary; this was to be the responsibility of Mr. Herbert Parsons, a White philanthropist interested in Blacks' health. And, second, she was to be hired on an experimental basis, for two months only.

The nurse they chose was Jessie Sleet, who had been trained at the Provident Hospital in Chicago, a hospital for Black patients with a nurses' training school for Black women.[6] Having been told that the tuberculosis committee had not wanted to hire her and that her employment was temporary, Jessie Sleet accepted, with reservations, the position of district nurse with the COS on 3 October 1900.

"A Successful Experiment" was a news item that appeared in the first volume of the *American Journal of Nursing* in 1901. This article was unusual, especially for this time period, and contained a report written by Sleet for the COS describing her community health work among Black immigrants in New York:

> I beg to render to you a report of the work done by me as district nurse among the colored people of New York City during the months of October and November. I have endeavored to search out families in which there was sickness and destitution. But I have never hesitated to visit anyone when I have felt that a word of advice or a friendly warning was all they needed.
>
> I have visited forty-one sick families and made one hundred and fifty-six calls in connection with these families, caring for nine cases of consumption, four cases of peritonitis, two cases of chicken pox, two cases of cancer, one case of diphtheria, two cases of heart disease, two cases of tumor, one case of gastric catarrh, two cases of pneumonia, four cases of rheumatism, and two cases of scalp-wound.
>
> I have given baths, applied poultices, dressed wounds, washed and dressed new-born babes, cared for mothers. When there has been an intelligent member of the family on whom I could depend, I have instructed them how to care for the sick one. When there was not one, as was often the case, I have made daily visits if the case required it, caring for them until they were able to care for

themselves. Whenever I have felt it advisable, I have urged them to go into hospitals.

Sleet then describes in detail two cases that interested her greatly and for which she obtained good results. The following excerpt is from the second case:

> B—— S——, a consumptive, twenty-seven years of age, with no means of support, a little girl of three years, and a mother sixty-five, lived in three small rooms. . . . The three persons occupied the one room and slept in the same bed, the sick woman refusing to be separated from her child for a few hours. After I had visited the family a few times I succeeded in convincing the mother that she was endangering the life of her child. On my advice, she agreed to occupy the room alone, permitting the others to sleep in another apartment. A marked improvement was noticeable in other directions. The sputum was always carefully covered and a window lowered from the top whenever the weather permitted. The mother of the sick girl did not ask for relief, but that assistance be given her in obtaining work. I was successful in finding her work for ten days to do house-cleaning. The lady became interested in the family, and procured for the daughter the services of a specialist, who gave her every attention. The mother earned sufficient to pay a month's rent which was over-due, thus keeping her little home together, which was on the verge of going to pieces. The daughter, who passed away a few days ago, was made comfortable up to the day of her death.[7]

Jessie Sleet performed her duties so well that after a year she was given a permanent position with the organization.[8] Sleet became a legendary figure in the field of community health nursing and paved the way for Black nurses to practice in the community health nursing field. She is credited with providing district nursing care to hundreds and was instrumental in persuading more Black patients to seek nursing and medical care.

Elizabeth Tyler: Innovator and Community Nursing Health Care Reformer

In 1906, Lillian D. Wald, founder and director of the Henry Street Settlement Visiting Nursing Service, heard of Sleet's success at the COS and asked her to recommend a Black nurse for her organization. Jessie Sleet recommended Miss Elizabeth Tyler, a schoolmate and graduate of Freedmen's Hospital Training School for Nurses in Washington, D.C.[9] Freedmen's[10] was established in 1894 for the sole purpose of training Black

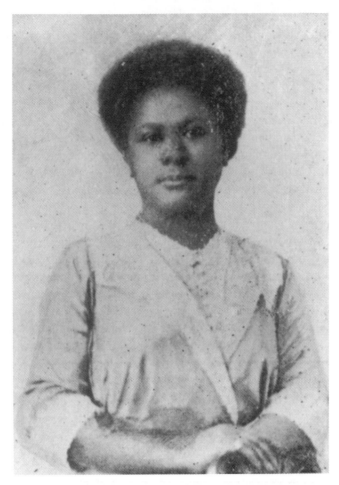

Figure 2. Elizabeth Tyler. (By permission of Dr. M. Elizabeth Carnegie)

women who were interested in becoming nurses. Applicants had first to work under the supervision of the superintendent of nurses at Freedmen's Hospital, who determined if applicants were physically and psychologically suited for the profession. After working for an undetermined amount of time and obtaining the superintendent's approval, the young women were tentatively accepted into the training school and served a probation period of one month, during which all applicants were also given pre-tests in reading, penmanship, English diction, and arithmetic. After completion of

all of the screening procedures, applicants were then officially admitted into the program; admission took place at any time during the year, whenever there was a vacancy.

On 15 November 1894, Freedmen's received its first students, and thirty-seven young women, including Elizabeth Tyler, embarked upon life-long and rewarding careers. The course of study at Freedmen's was not easy. As was the case in so many other nurses' training schools in the country at the time, student nurses constituted Freedmen's primary labor force. During the first nine months of training, Tyler and her classmates served as assistants on the wards of Freedmen's Hospital. Along with providing care to assigned patients, their duties included cleaning, meal preparations, and staff relief. They worked around the clock with very little free time for recreation. When they were not actively involved in practical work on the wards, the students had to attend lectures and recitations. During the second nine months of their training, the students were required to perform any duties assigned them by the superintendent of nurses. These assignments covered the full range of responsibilities usually assumed by nurses who had already graduated. Ward work, charge nurse assignments, staffing and relief responsibilities, and private duty nursing assignments were just a few of the types of jobs performed by Tyler and her classmates. When assigned as private duty nurses, these students, although unsupervised, were responsible for providing total care for patients, be they rich or poor, in their homes throughout the Washington area.

After graduating from Freedmen's, Tyler left Washington and sought employment in the surrounding states. The only job offered her was in private duty nursing. Tyler, like the other Black nurses of her time, was primarily confined to providing care to members of her own race and a limited number of White patients. The best assignments, however, usually went to White nurses who worked through hospital registries. Since few Black people could afford the fees for private duty nurses, little work was available for Black nurses. The only other positions available for Black nurses were those in general duty nursing for Blacks in hospitals that admitted prescribed quotas of Black patients. These positions were also scarce, since much of the hospital care was given by pupil nurses. Tyler settled for employment as a private duty nurse in Northampton, Massachusetts.[11] Here her patient caseload was limited mainly to students enrolled at Smith College,[12] and after two years Tyler decided that this experience was neither financially nor professionally rewarding. Hearing of job possibilities in Alabama through other Black nurses, she left Massachusetts and went south.

After her arrival in Alabama, Tyler initially appeared to be in another job maze, and she was not quite sure what she wanted to do; but she was relatively sure she no longer wanted to work as a private duty nurse. When the opening for a resident nurse at A&M College in Normal, Alabama, was announced, Tyler immediately applied and was hired. In addition to her responsibilities as resident nurse at A&M, Tyler taught physiology and hygiene.[13] She so thoroughly enjoyed this kind of nursing that when an opening of the same type was offered in Virginia, she resigned her position at A&M and assumed the same responsibilities at St. Paul Normal and Industrial School in Lawrenceville, where she worked for two years. Although she was very happy with this job, she wanted to continue her education and experience in other areas of nursing. When she heard about the postgraduate course offered at Lincoln School for Nurses in New York City (which had been inspired by Adah B. Thoms, a Lincoln graduate and the school's only Black nursing supervisor), she resigned her position in Lawrenceville and moved to New York.

Shortly after her arrival in New York City, Tyler learned of the possibility for employment in the area of community health nursing. In need of employment as well as desiring an education, she applied to the Henry Street Settlement for a position as a visiting health nurse and, in addition, enrolled in the postgraduate course in general nursing at Lincoln. In 1906, Tyler became the first Black Henry Street Settlement visiting nurse.

Tyler's job as a Henry Street nurse would not be as rewarding as she had at first believed, nor would it be an easy one. Because there were no Black patients at Henry Street, Tyler began to ask apartment house janitors if they knew of any cases of illness among the Black tenants in their buildings. Although she had a difficult time at first convincing the janitors that she did not have anything to sell and was not an intruder, she finally gained their confidence and was permitted to go through the buildings to make friendly visits to the tenants. After three months, she had acquired enough patients to require the assistance of a second nurse.[14] Tyler reported her progress among the Black people in her district to Lillian Wald and informed her that she would need another nurse to assist her. The nurse sent to help Tyler was Edith Carter, the second Black nurse hired by Henry Street. (Carter's life and career will be described in more detail below.)[15]

STILLMAN HOUSE: A SETTLEMENT HOUSE FOR BLACKS

A news item in the September 1906 issue of the *American Journal of Nursing* reported,

From Miss Dock we learn that the Nurses' Settlement in New York is happy in several important additions to its work. A most gratifying and needed extension in the Visiting Nursing Service has been made in an upper west side region where the colored people live. Salaries have been given for two nurses who are also colored and who have settled in their district in a flat. The work is fortunate indeed in the rare ability and devotion of these two women, Miss Tyler and Miss Carter. . . . Beside being excellent nurses, they are both especially alive to social movement organized preventive work.[16]

In December 1906, Elizabeth Tyler established the Stillman House Branch of the Henry Street Settlement for Colored People in a small store on West 61st Street. Stillman House was one of several outreach houses throughout the city under the Henry Street Settlement organization. Tyler hoped that this work would grow and become as important to San Juan Hill as the work of Henry Street Settlement was to the Lower East Side.[17]

SAN JUAN HILL

Located in the borough of Manhattan on the West Side of New York City, San Juan Hill (now known as Columbus Hill) was the most congested, disease-ridden community in the city. Bounded by 54th Street on the south, 70th Street on the north, Central Park West and Eighth Avenue on the east, and the Hudson River on the west, this teeming community encompassed fifty-five city blocks and housed thousands of native Whites, Jews, Irish, Italians, and Blacks. San Juan Hill, like other communities in the city, had quiet and attractive neighborhoods, but the section where Blacks lived was the most severely congested section of the area. Large numbers of Blacks lived mostly on one street: West 61st Street.

On the lower end of West 61st Street was an area of two and a half acres that contained 1,641 Blacks. West 61st Street and the areas surrounding it were so heavily populated that the New York Department of Health divided it in half and designated it as Sanitary Areas 47 and 51.[18] Eighty percent of the entire San Juan Hill Black population lived in these areas; more than half were foreign born. In 1922, 5,861 Blacks hailed from the West Indies, while the remaining 2,048 came from Central America, Cuba, and South America. Each of these groups of foreign Blacks strove to maintain their cultural heritage and ethnic beliefs, as did their Jewish, Italian, and Irish neighbors.

The settlement of foreign-born Blacks in San Juan Hill added another complication to existing racial problems in this ethnically diverse and divided community. For years, San Juan Hill had been known for infighting

among Blacks and Whites; now it was also known as a community where Blacks were pitted against Blacks. There were regular clashes between one group or another (in fact, the district was satirically called San Juan Hill because fighting among all of the races was so common); however, conflicts between Blacks and the Irish were the most frequent. The antagonism between these two groups was undoubtedly one of the harshest intergroup hatreds in American history. Blacks born in the United States often expressed their dislike of foreigners, Black or White, and of the Irish in particular.

Such statements as "In this land of Bibles where the outcasts — the scum of European society — can come and enjoy the fullest social and political privileges, the Native Born American with wooly hair and dark complexion is made the victim . . . of Social Ostracism . . . " and "Tens of thousand of aliens are being landed on these shores and freely given the employment which is denied the Negro citizens . . . " and "The time is upon us when some of the restriction will have to be placed upon the volume and character of European immigration . . . " could be read in *The New York Age, The Crisis,* and *The New York Freeman.*[19] Throughout the nineteenth century, this mutual antipathy erupted into violence many times, leading to numerous deaths among the Irish and the Blacks.

Notwithstanding the racial and ethnic conflict, the growing numbers of deaths among Blacks in San Juan Hill were also a result of the relative lack of medical care offered by the medical establishment and ineffective responses to the all-too-frequent epidemics of disease. In the second decade of the twentieth century, the death rate per 100,000 Blacks of all ages in the San Juan Hill district was 5,255. The most prevalent causes of death were tuberculosis (544 per 100,000), pneumonia (561 per 100,000), heart disease (412 per 100,000), and diarrhea (168 per 100,000). The infant mortality rate in the district stood at 255 per 100,000, and the most prevalent causes of death were diarrhea, congenital debility, and respiratory disease.[20]

Initially, the opportunity for Black community health nurses to serve this heretofore unserved population was made possible entirely through the generosity of Mrs. Edward Harkness and her sister, Miss Charlotte Stillman, who provided funds for nurses' salaries, office rents, supplies, and, later, rent for nurses' apartments in the neighborhood. Mrs. Harkness and Miss Stillman's act of kindness to the Blacks on New York's West Side, it is said, was an expression of gratitude to a Black nanny who had cared for them throughout most of their childhood.

When Tyler and Carter requested assignment to the San Juan Hill

district, they assumed the responsibility for the care of all the Black people residing on Manhattan's West Side.[21] Their district included several other Black neighborhoods in addition to San Juan Hill. Realizing the vastness of their work, the two nurses decided to divide the district in half, with Tyler covering the area from 62nd Street to Harlem and Carter covering the area from 61st Street to the Battery. The nurses were not immediately well received by the Black people in their district. Despite the fact that they too were Black, Tyler and Carter's presence represented an unrequested intrusion by the White establishment and they were therefore viewed with fear and mistrust. Tyler and Carter visited doctors' offices to seek their assistance and visited churches to look at the "tablets" to see who was sick in the congregation; they followed people who were obviously ill to their homes and tried to convince them to accept help. Much persuasion was needed to gain entry into Blacks' homes. However, once these patients and potential patients accepted the two nurses, they were treated as friends and were graciously received into their homes.

Faced with rampant disease, neglect, ignorance, and the prevailing racial tension, Tyler and Carter confronted a tremendous amount of work. They spent their days in unsafe, dirty, disease-ridden, and congested neighborhoods. Moving purposefully in and out of dingy, overcrowded houses described as "human hives, honeycombed with rooms thick with human beings,"[22] these courageous, self-assured women assumed the monumental task of providing physical comfort, psychological support, health education, and bedside care to thousands of Black infants, children, men and women.

Tyler and Carter not only concerned themselves with the social, economic, and political environment, which bore directly on high mortality rates among Blacks in their district, they also contended with a multitude of traditional cures, including potions, deliverance, exorcism, physical healing, herbs and roots, and superstitions associated with each of the different groups of Blacks they served. So many different beliefs about illness and other social and health-related issues in such close proximity greatly affected the population's health and posed a major problem for public officials.

In addition, the two nurses often had to compete with local quacks who guaranteed they could purge their patients of every imaginable ailment.[23] Reliance on quackery and medical superstition played a more harmful role in Black social life than it did for any other minority group.[24] Determined to serve and save as many people as they could, Tyler and Carter were on a mission that, given its scope and complexity, was a distinct work of faith.

THE WORK CONTINUES: MORE CONTRIBUTIONS BY ELIZABETH TYLER

In 1914, nine years after her career as a Henry Street nurse began, Tyler, confident that the work at Stillman House was well established, resigned and moved to Philadelphia. The Henry Phipps Institute was the primary treatment facility in Philadelphia for Blacks who were afflicted with tuber- culosis. It was located in the center of the city's Black community. Despite the fact that Phipps was in a convenient location and that large numbers of Blacks in this area were infected with the disease, few availed themselves of the services offered. Prior to Tyler's employment at Phipps, the facility treated fewer than 100 patients annually. Blacks in Philadelphia, like those in New York, feared and distrusted the medical establishment and all those affiliated with it, be they Black or White. Tyler set in motion a patient recruitment campaign similar to the one she and Carter used when they established Stillman House. So successful was she that by the time she left the institute in 1921, the number of patients treated annually had grown from 100 to 3,000.

After Tyler resigned from Phipps, she became the first Black nurse to be employed by the State Health and Welfare Commission of Delaware. Her responsibilities at this agency were to organize and take charge of the child hygiene work for the state. Under Tyler's leadership, well-baby and tuberculosis clinics were established. After her work in Delaware was well established and a permanent and competent staff in place, Tyler resigned her position and went to New Jersey, where she accepted a job in Newark with the New Jersey Tuberculosis League (a position very similar to the one she had held in Delaware). Tyler was the first Black nurse to be employed there. For the next three and a half years, she developed educational pro- grams geared to the health needs of Blacks at the local and state levels. When she left this position, Tyler next moved to the Essex County Tuber- culosis League in Newark, where she continued to provide health educa- tion for New Jersey's Black population. So successful was her work, that the state closed the state Black health education department and transferred its work to the Essex County Tuberculosis League.

Edith M. Carter: Satisfied to Carry the Bag

Edith M. Carter was born on 17 April 1865 in New Rochelle, New York.[25] Growing up there, Carter, like most young women of any race, was taught to be a homemaker. She was expected to remain with or close to her family, and was never encouraged to go off into the world to become a professional

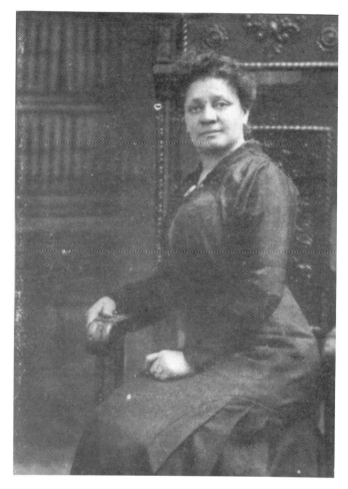

Figure 3. Edith Carter. (By permission of Visiting Nurse Service of New York)

worker. She was also expected to find a suitable young man, marry, have children, and settle into a life much like that of her mother. Following the social norms, Carter did remain at home, close to her family; however, she never married or had any children.

It is not known if caring for her ailing mother for so many years was her motivation to choose nursing as a career; but what is known is that after the death of her mother and after consulting her minister,[26] Carter, at the age of thirty-one, entered nurses' training at Freedmen's Hospital School of

Nursing in 1896. In 1898, she earned her nursing diploma and returned to her family in New Rochelle. During the next eight years she worked in a hospital owned by one of the most prominent physicians in town, who had known her since childhood.

In the spring of 1906, Carter went to the Henry Street Settlement for a job interview, and on May 6 of the same year she was hired. She left New Rochelle and her work in the hospital when she heard of the work being done by Lillian Wald and her staff at the Settlement House on Henry Street. The Henry Street Settlement Visiting Nurse Service hired her and assigned her to work with Elizabeth Tyler in San Juan Hill.

Being a dedicated nurse and truly caring about the people she served, Carter fought for them, believed in them, and nursed them when others had given them up. In one case, a doctor had done all that he could for a patient, and still she showed no progress. He felt that the patient was beyond help, and so gave Carter permission to do whatever she wished to provide the patient comfort. Under her care, the patient's ulcers, which were the cause of her poor prognosis, healed and she recovered. Another patient, who had been in the hospital for weeks fighting what appeared to be a losing battle against pneumonia, had become emaciated and had developed such huge infected decubitus ulcers that she was sent home to die. When Carter arrived at her home, the neighbors were standing helplessly outside her door. Again, under the nurse's care the ulcers were healed and the patient not only recovered, she later gave birth to two babies.[27]

Carter describes a third successful intervention in a summary of patients she cared for in November 1916:

> I have been interested in the care of Jessie N—— . . . This poor woman had two children ages 3 years — 18 mo. and the baby of three mo. who had never gained an ounce since birth, died in Oct. The family was supported by her aged mother as the husband was worthless, and living away from home. When the mother could spare a dollar she would stop on her way home from work and ask the Dr. to come and see Jessie. The last time he called, he told her not to send for him again until she had six dollars, when he would bring an assistant and tap the Pt. This was the second Dr. called to the case — the first gave a diagnosis of uterine cancer and Pul T.B. He afterward said the sputum was neg. The sec. physician gave Brights. Had tried to persuade Pt. to call a Dr. from Van. Clinic, but they feared that he would only send her to Bellevue where she had been during the month of Sept. and came home rather than be transferred to the Island.[28]

Carter continued to work with Jessie despite the fact that the medical establishment considered her noncompliant and had given up on her. Ac-

cording to Carter's progress notes, she finally convinced Jessie to accept medical care and convinced an institution to accept her. Jessie was referred to Vanderbilt Clinic, where she received free medical treatment. Having taken care of Jessie's immediate problem, Carter informed the Social Service Department at Vanderbilt about the family's situation. Through Carter's persistent efforts, Jessie and her family were able to receive groceries and bed linens free of charge. The mother was given $4.50 per week so that she might spend more time at home with her daughter. The husband was given work temporarily and he was made to contribute to the family. In addition, Dr. Schulman of the Vanderbilt Clinic visited Jessie on an outpatient basis every other day and her medicine was furnished free from the dispensary. Because of Carter's commitment to her patient's well-being, Jessie recovered from her illness and was discharged, cured by Vanderbilt and Henry Street. In addition to the care provided to Jessie and her family during November of 1916, Carter made 185 nursing visits, 51 substitution visits, and 8 social service visits.[29]

Edith Carter gained much notoriety among the patients she served in San Juan Hill. According to Dorothy Cooper, supervisor of the Longacre Office of the Henry Street Visiting Nurse Service:

> To the people in this area Miss Carter *is* Henry Street. She is a welcome friend to all who live there and to walk through this district with her makes you wonder how she ever gets to the homes to visit cases, for she is stopped every other step to give advice to some mother, talk to a child, or to pass the time of day with some old friend who is so glad to see her nurse. Families wait on their doorsteps to see Miss Carter as she comes down the block so they can ask her to call on a sick friend or member of their family. . . .
>
> To Miss Carter the area is just one large family she is happy to serve as their nurse. To the families Miss Carter is "Their Henry Street Nurse" and the friend to whom they can take all their problems knowing that she will somehow help them find a satisfactory solution. . . .
>
> Miss Carter's twenty-eight years [*sic*] experience give to one a picture of the development of Visiting Nursing. When she came to the organization, she was given her bag and appointed to the area in which she was to work and instructed to visit Doctors, Ministers, Clinics, and the Janitors to find out who was ill in the homes and needed her care. She lived in the district so that families could come to her apartment for consultation. Once a week down to Henry Street Settlement to have her records supervised and to discuss the families she was visiting. To the nurse who comes to Henry Street today for experience her introduction to our field is carefully planned and supervised and Miss Carter is always a help to the younger nurse. To have seen and to have been a part of the growth of this organization from one to twenty-one offices

and from about twenty-five nurses to two hundred nurses is an experience we all envy. [Emphasis in original.][30]

Conclusion

Jessie Sleet, Elizabeth Tyler, and Edith Carter, pioneers in community health nursing in New York City, began their work during a period of industrialization, immigration, and great population growth in the midst of teeming slums, disease, and death. For Blacks, it was a time of change, turmoil, deplorable living and health conditions, and extremely high death rates among individuals of all ages. For community health nursing, it was a time of establishment, activism, expansion, and development. And for these Black community health nurse pioneers, it was a time of tremendous challenges and growth.

Confronted with pervasive ignorance and superstitions among culturally diverse Blacks, Black community health nurses serving in New York City had to struggle unrelentingly to correct harmful and deadly practices while attempting to render health care to their patients. Hindered also by educational, professional, and racial barriers, and confronted with increasing mortality among people of their race, Sleet, Tyler, and Carter found creative ways to transcend these barriers and overcome the circumstances that restricted their practices and destroyed their patients' lives.

MARIE O. PITTS MOSLEY, EdD, RN
Assistant Professor
Bellevue School of Nursing
Hunter College
425 East Twenty-fifth Street
New York, N.Y. 10010
Phone: (212) 481-7574

Notes

1. Mabel Keaton Staupers, *No Time for Prejudice: A Story of the Integration of Negroes in Nursing in the United States* (New York: Macmillan, 1961), 7; Adah B. Thoms, *Pathfinders: A History of the Progress of Colored Graduate Nurses* (New York: Kay Printing House, 1929), 9; Mary Roberts, *American Nursing: History and Interpretation* (New York: Macmillan, 1955), 56.

2. Mary Elizabeth Carnegie, *The Path We Tread: Blacks in Nursing, 1854–1984* (New York: J. B. Lippincott, 1986), 146.

3. "Nurses' Settlement News," *American Journal of Nursing* 6 (September 1906): 832–33 (hereafter cited as *AJN*); Lavinia L. Dock, *A History of Nursing from the Earliest Time to the Present Day with Special Reference to the Work of the Past Thirty Years* (New York: G. P. Putnam's Sons, 1912), 3:104.

4. "Nurses' Settlement News," *AJN*, 832–33.

5. Staupers, 7.

6. Ulysses Grant Dailey, "Daniel Hale Williams: Pioneer Surgeon and Father of Negro Hospitals" (paper delivered at meeting of the National Hospital Association, Chicago, 18 August 1941, mimeographed at Providence Hospital and Training School), 1.

7. Lucy L. Drown, "A Successful Experiment," *AJN* 1, no. 10 (July 1901): 729–31.

8. Drown, 729–31. For additional discussion relative to Miss Sleet's employment as a district nurse in New York City, see Marie O. Pitts Mosley, "Jessie Sleet Scales: First Black Public Health Nurse," *ABNF Journal* 5, no. 2 (March/April 1994): 45–51; Mosley, "A History of Black Leaders in Nursing: The Influence of Four Black Community Health Nurses on the Establishment, Growth, and Practice of Public Health Nursing in New York City, 1906–1930" (PhD diss., Teachers College, Columbia University, 1992), 72–98; Anna B. Coles, "The Howard University School of Nursing in Historical Perspective," *Journal of the National Medical Association* 61, no. 2 (March 1969): 105; Joyce Ann Elmore, "Black Nurses: Their Service and Their Struggle," *AJN* 76, no. 3 (March 1976): 436; Staupers, 47; Thoms, 15–17.

9. Carnegie, 146.

10. For additional information on the Freedmen's Hospital Training School for Nurses, see Elmore, "A History of Freedmen's Hospital Training School for Nursing in Washington, D.C., 1894–1901" (Master's thesis, Catholic University, 1965).

11. Thoms, 40.

12. Ibid.

13. Ibid.

14. Ibid., 41.

15. Minutes of Semiannual Meeting of the Board of Directors, 1 May 1907, Visiting Nurse Service Archives; "Nurses' Settlement News," *AJN*, 832; Coles, 107; Carnegie, 149; Thoms, 44.

16. "Nurses' Settlement News," *AJN*, 832.

17. Thoms, 41.

18. During the late nineteenth and early twentieth centuries, in order to provide the most accurate illness and disease statistical information to New York City health officials, Dr. Walter Laidlaw, a statistician, developed a disease inventory system designed to allow health officials to plan for the provision of health services, both under public and private leadership in all branches of health work. The Laidlaw system divided and subdivided already existing health districts into smaller, more contained health districts called *sanitary areas*. Using statistical information

such as that provided by Dr. Laidlaw, health officials could pinpoint conditions that were peculiar to particular areas in order to dictate the types and amounts of health care resources needed.

19. For more discussions on the interracial conflicts between Blacks and the Irish in New York City, see *The Crisis* 12 (August 1917): 166–67; *The New York Freeman*, 15 May 1886; *The New York Age*, 25 May 1905 and 5 October 1916.

20. Summary of Negro Population in Columbus Hill and Vicinity, 1910 and 1920, Lillian D. Wald Collection, Rare Books and Manuscript Library, Butler Library, Columbia University, New York, box 45, folder: "Summary of Negro Population." Information found in this document discusses the population, racial classes, housing, and mortality statistics in the Columbus Hill District for 1910 and 1920. For additional health statistical information on this district, see also Report of Dependent Negro Families Under A.I.C.P. Care, Fiscal Year 1926–1927, Community Service Society, Rare Books and Manuscript Library, Butler Library, box 36, folder: "Study of 336 Dependent Negro Families"; General Director to Mr. Franklin B. Kirkbride, 13 January 1917, 11 April 1917, and 5 February 1918, Butler Library; and L. Hollingworth Wood of the National League on Urban Conditions among Negroes to Mr. Franklin P. Kirkbride, 7 March 1917, Butler Library.

21. The nursing care provided by Tyler and Carter was primarily for Blacks residing in their district. They did provide care to Whites in the district, but only in cases of emergency. The reason for this segregated nursing care was related to the special interest of the Stillman family. Additionally, Tyler and Carter, wishing to work with members of their own race, requested a health district with large numbers of unserved Blacks, an area whose numbers would keep them extremely busy. For additional discussion about the racial background of patients cared for by Tyler and Carter in their district can be found in Lillian D. Wald's Report of the Henry Street (Nurses') Settlement, 17 March 1909, Visiting Nurse Service of New York Archives.

22. Mary White Ovington, *Half a Man: The Status of the Negro in New York* (New York: Hill and Wang, 1969): 22.

23. *The New York Globe*, 16 February 1884.

24. Gilbert Osofsky, *Harlem: The Making of a Ghetto* (New York: Harper & Row, 1966), 9.

25. Date and place of birth are contained in file letters located at the Visiting Nursing Service of New York Archives.

26. Information extracted from "File Letter," Visiting Nursing Service of New York Archives.

27. Dorothy Elizabeth Jensen, "The Henry Street Settlement: A Response to the Needs of the Sick Poor, 1893–1913" (PhD diss., Teachers College, Columbia University, 1979), 130.

28. The "Island" referred to in this document was Ward Island, located on New York City's East River adjacent to the Island of Manhattan. Patients infected with tuberculosis were sent there for treatment and cure. Black patients, however, were particularly afraid of being sent there because it was viewed as a place where one went to die; they would only consent to admission when home remedies, religious interventions, or culturally derived approaches failed to provide cures, or

when health officials forced them to go. From Edith M. Carter's summary of Stillman for the month of November 1916 (entry dated 10 December 1916), addressed to Bessie Ely Amerman, RN, superintendent of nurses at the Henry Street Settlement, document located at Visiting Nurse Service of New York Archives.

29. Carter, summary of Stillman for the month of November 1916.

30. Dorothy Cooper, supervisor of the Longacre Office of the Henry Street Settlement Visiting Nurse Service, "Longacre," Visiting Nursing Service of New York Archives.

The Origins of Modern Nursing in the Netherlands

Nanny Wiegman
Department of Medical History
Free University, Amsterdam

Introduction

In the historiography of nursing, the hospital-trained nurse is often treated as the final stage in the development of modern nursing. Originally women's work for family, friends, and community, nursing was augmented in the nineteenth century with a great variety of aims and forms, religious as well as lay. In the second half of the century, medical developments and reforms in poor law systems, combined with complex social, economic, and political factors, created new standards for nursing. One focal point was the modern hospital, where nurse training and practice were offered, improved, and standardized. Over time, nursing skill came to be defined as the acquisition of specific training formally recognized by a certificate from a reputable hospital. According to Morris Vogel, the modern hospital became the source of the "best" medical care, rendering more traditional sites of care obsolete. Due to great changes in the organization of social, economic, and urban life, patients opted to enter hospitals for a variety of nonmedical reasons.[1]

Though nursing the sick is universal, nursing has evolved with many national variations. Although the modern professional nurse was slow to take shape, the process of orienting nursing toward the hospital was already well under way in England by the 1860s.[2] By the turn of the century, almost half of all nurses worked in general hospitals. Of these, three-quarters were nurses in training and a quarter were qualified, well-trained nurses.[3]

In the Netherlands, however, the modern hospital, characterized by the admission of patients of all social classes and the existence of a formal hospital-based nurse training system, took much longer to emerge. Dutch

Nursing History Review 4 (1996): 83–97. Copyright © 1996 by The American Association for the History of Nursing.

hospitals took shape very slowly in the last part of the nineteenth century; hospital-based nurse training became widely accepted only after 1910. In this article I want to analyze Dutch developments in nursing from a comparative perspective, taking England as a rival model.[4] I will first explain the timing of health care developments in the Netherlands. Second, I will discuss the character of nineteenth-century care in the Netherlands, showing that Dutch nursing in this period was very well adapted to Dutch socioeconomic and religious circumstances. Finally, I will sketch the emergence of the modern hospital-trained Dutch nurse.[5]

Factors Affecting the Late Development of Dutch Hospital-Based Nursing

Nursing historians seem to agree on the important influence of war, colonization, and industrialization and urbanization on shaping nursing in the nineteenth century. In the Netherlands at that time, these influences were lacking.

War tends to stimulate the development of surgical care, but only in the 1850s did nursing of wounded military personnel become a subject of public debate. As Anne Summers has argued in *Angels and Citizens,* it was only when war became more of a civilian concern that women became involved.[6] In an age of nationalism, when recruitment for the military was not limited to social outcasts and when enlistment was seen as a national duty, women who organized hospitals and took care of the wounded began to be regarded as national heroines. In English history, the Crimean War was such a turning point. The extensive news coverage of the war and its terrible consequences for soldiers sparked a movement that advocated improving medical care and including women in the nursing of wounded soldiers.

Between the end of the Napoleonic Wars in 1815 and the German invasion in 1940, however, there was peace in the Netherlands. Even during the Revolution of 1830, when the Belgians broke away from the Kingdom of the Netherlands to found their own state, there were only a few skirmishes. The Dutch, who had achieved the status of a world power in the seventeenth century, successfully adapted themselves to the role of a small but independent state in the nineteenth century. Dutch foreign policy was characterized by the evasion of war and the safeguarding of the country's

neutrality. International cooperation based on a system of international law became the cornerstone of foreign policy.[7] In this climate, military expenditure was frowned upon and the development of military medicine came to a halt; students did not see the variety of diseases and wounds found especially in war conditions, and Dutch military medical education after 1865 declined in quality.[8]

The absence of war inhibited the development of military nursing. The vicissitudes of the Dutch branch of the International Red Cross illustrate this. Founded in 1867, the Dutch Red Cross soon had support from many women's societies engaged in organizing nurse training. However, though student nurses were occasionally allowed to work in hospitals to improve their practical skills, they met the same problem student military surgeons encountered, a lack of war-inflicted wounds. Although various local departments of the Dutch Red Cross continued to educate nurses who could pass a theoretical examination, the nurses had little chance to practice. Dutch Red Cross nurses found their first and only chance to build up practical experience on foreign soil during the Franco-German War of 1870–1871.[9]

Colonial imperialism also stimulated the broadening of nurse training in Britain. The British colonial wars of the second half of the nineteenth century in India and Africa were part of an extended scheme of imperial expansion and provided the first test of the Army Nursing Service.[10] Such stimuli were absent in the Netherlands, even though, traditionally, the Netherlands was a more important colonial power. As far as imperialism was concerned, the Dutch attitude was paradoxical.[11] With regard to the economic exploitation of their colonies, they were virtually unrivaled, but they did not follow a policy of formal expansion through war. The Dutch military medical service in the East Indies mirrored this state of affairs; designed in 1817, it remained unchanged throughout the nineteenth century.[12]

However, during the last decades of the nineteenth century, Dutch policy began to change. Although not imperialist in the strict sense of the word, the Netherlands would not tolerate any foreign competition in the Dutch East Indies and began to subdue the whole territory. Initially, the wars with indigenous rulers had little impact in the motherland. The Dutch kept the East Indian Army separate from its domestic army and recruited its personnel mostly from a European reservoir of social outcasts.[13] Because of this policy, war casualties at first had little influence on public opinion. Only in the 1880s, in the last phase of the Atjeh War (Atjeh was one of the last

territories that had to be subdued), did changes in military recruitment make the sacrifice of human lives in colonial wars a public issue. This resulted in some improvements in military medicine in the colonies.[14]

Thus, during the nineteenth century, military and colonial developments had little impact on Dutch nursing. However, the slow rate of industrialization in the Netherlands had an even more decisive effect on hospital development. The transformation of the traditional hospital to its modern equivalent is rarely thought by historians to be dependent on medical improvements alone. Nonmedical factors, such as fundamental changes in the social fabric of urban life, are now recognized to be of great importance as well. The emergence of an industrial society created a whole new set of circumstances in which hospital care came to be an attractive or even necessary alternative to home nursing by relatives. Physically confined living conditions in the hastily erected buildings of rapidly urbanizing cities made home nursing more difficult. Just as important was the distance of the patients' workplace from their homes and the anxiety employers had concerning sick employees as a source of contagious diseases. Many new workers in industrial areas were isolated from home and family, leading to acceptance of hospitalization during sickness.[15]

By the middle of the nineteenth century, industrialization was well under way in most of Europe. However, the Netherlands remained a nonindustrial society with traditional production methods until the beginning of the twentieth century. Only after 1870, albeit still on a limited scale, did traditional patterns change. In the 1890s, there was a real industrial takeoff, which within a few decades brought the Netherlands to an industrial level similar to that of neighboring countries.[16]

Due to their slow industrial development, the Dutch were late in urbanizing. This does not mean, however, that the Netherlands should be regarded as a rural country. At the end of the seventeenth century, about 60 percent of the population lived in numerous small but economically important towns in the coastal provinces of Holland. Until late in the nineteenth century, this pattern hardly changed. Amsterdam, for instance, by far the largest city in the Netherlands, had 180,000 inhabitants at the beginning of the nineteenth century, and it was only after 1870 that it began to expand.[17] New cities, a phenomenon so typical of modern industrial areas such as the Midlands in Britain, were also absent from the Netherlands.

Thus, the high level of Dutch urbanization, especially in the coastal regions, dated from the middle of the seventeenth century when the Netherlands was a world economic power. These "early modern" cities were

characterized by a high degree of social organization and an extended network of public services. Widows, orphans, the homeless, and the aged were relatively well taken care of. Church agencies, supported by private charity, provided most of the financial support, while local authorities made up the rest.[18] The care of the sick was closely connected to this urban system of poor relief. Every town, big or small, had at least one or more *gasthuis* (traditional hospital) at its disposal where the poor and the aged could be given shelter and, in cases of illness, some limited forms of nursing care. In larger cities, these traditional hospitals were often funded by local government. In towns with a university, these poor relief institutions also functioned as teaching hospitals.[19]

Such patterns of social and medical care can hardly be described as particular to the Netherlands. However, what kept Dutch developments distinct was the degree to which these traditional social organizations remained intact and impervious to change, right up to the end of the nineteenth century. The growing importance of government, both local and national, brought about fundamental changes in the organization of social and poor relief.[20] Religious poor relief organizations had to bow to the rules various government agencies imposed upon them and, after 1854, had to compete with a new municipal poor relief system. However, because hospitalization of the sick cost much more than home nursing, most poor relief agencies, religious as well as civic, opposed the extension or modernization of traditional hospitals.[21]

Nevertheless, at the end of the nineteenth century, the system began to change, but only in a few big cities such as Amsterdam and Rotterdam. Some traditional hospitals were modernized by reformist physicians and new hospitals based on new medical needs were also founded, but the physicians had to work within the stringent conditions set down by parsimonious poor relief agencies.[22]

Socioeconomic and Religious Circumstances of Dutch Nursing in the Nineteenth Century

Although Dutch hospital nursing emerged later than in other countries, this does not imply that the Dutch were not interested in nursing developments elsewhere or that no new initiatives were taken. Foreign developments were discussed in the medical journals, but in the light of the Dutch situation. For example, in 1874, the Dutch physician Samuel Coronel

(1827–1892) justified his publishing of *Praktische Handleiding voor Zieken-verpleging* (Practical Manual for Nursing) by stressing the unsuitability of Nightingale's otherwise brilliant work, *Notes on Nursing,* for Dutch circumstances.[23] His approach was typical of that of the majority of nursing initiatives taken at that time, which were developed within the existing structures of local poor relief and philanthropy and adapted to a traditional society in which household, family, and community still played a central role. This resulted in a distinctive bias toward home nursing. Moreover, the development of Dutch nursing became intertwined in the religious rivalries that came to dominate the country's politics and culture.

In the 1830s, the Roman Catholics took the lead in implementing new nursing initiatives. Until 1798, the Catholics in the Netherlands had been treated as second-class citizens, especially in the coastal provinces, where they were a minority group. Only in the southern Netherlands had the Catholic system of primary education and poor relief remained intact.[24] From the 1820s onward, the Catholic church had tried to reinforce its institutional base in the northern Netherlands, and this policy had an important impact on nursing.

Amsterdam Catholics set an example in 1839 by asking the religious order Zusters van Liefde (Sisters of Love) to undertake home nursing. Central to this innovation was not the lack of space in the traditional hospitals, but the fear that Catholic souls might be tainted by a prolonged stay in a non-Catholic environment. The sisters did not receive any nurse training, but learned from one another in their work.[25] Although home nursing remained the nucleus of the order's work, a small facility was founded with a few beds for patients who for social reasons could not be nursed at home. No medical treatment was offered, and the organization conformed with the traditional hospital model. The sisters did not receive any pay, and the costs they incurred were financed from charity and poor relief funds.[26]

The Amsterdam initiative was a great success and became the model for similar institutions all over the country. Catholic congregational sisters lived in a rented building, often an annex to the home of the local priest, which was also the base for their home-nursing practice. These Catholic home-nursing institutions for the most part retained their link with the medical treatment offered by the traditional poor relief system.[27] The level of nurse training was limited but fully adapted to the services required.[28] However, when the modern hospital began to emerge, the lack of specialized nurse training for Catholic sisters was regarded as a problem, and remedies were discussed. The Onze Lieve Vrouwe Gasthuis (Our Holy

Virgin Hospital) in Amsterdam was the first Dutch Catholic institution to introduce a hospital-based training program for nurses in 1899. Eleven sisters received their nursing certificates two years later.[29] In 1910 the Onze Lieve Vrouwe Gasthuis was again a pioneer when it founded a similar program for lay nurses. These examples were soon followed in the smaller cities and in the countryside.[30]

Protestant nursing initiatives were also part of a religious mission program triggered by the success of the Catholic home-nursing campaign. Furthermore, from the 1830s on, the so-called Protestant Reveil Movement denounced the liberal theology reigning within the established Reformed Church and tried to find new ways of making Christianity work in day-to-day life. The care of the sick was one way of putting Christ's example into practice, especially for women. Protestant pastors took the initiative, and their missionary zeal, with a strong streak of anti-Catholicism, very much determined the development of Protestant nursing. The first orthodox Protestant initiative was the foundation of the Diaconessenhuis (Deaconess House) in Utrecht in 1844, modeled on the example set by Theodor Fliedner's deaconess movement in Germany.[31] At first the congregational organization of the deaconesses in the Netherlands met with severe criticism. For many opponents, it too much resembled the Catholic model they set out to oppose. Just like the Catholic deaconesses, they engaged in home nursing and brought a strong missionary flavor to their work. The nursing facilities they offered remained small and more often than not occupied part of the building needed for housing the deaconesses themselves. The Utrecht deaconesses did receive some formal training, but the leadership put an emphasis on subjects such as religion, singing, and calligraphy. In selecting new deaconesses, equal emphasis was placed on religious and nursing qualities.[32] At first the Utrecht Diaconessenhuis had limited success. Although the number of deaconesses gradually increased, it took twenty years before another deaconess congregation could be founded, and only after 1880 did the deaconess system put down firm roots in the Netherlands.[33] Although the deaconesses concentrated on home nursing, the strong religious flavor of their mission long stood in the way of the full deployment of their nursing experience. For example, the Utrecht foundation witnessed a prolonged debate on the question of whether home nursing or missionary work should be the institution's primary goal.

Liberal Protestantism also took its share of the burden of home nursing. In 1843 a group of liberal doctors and philanthropists founded the Vereeniging voor Ziekenverpleging (Society for Sick Nursing) in Amster-

dam.[34] There were various motives behind this foundation. On the one hand, the society wanted to spread civic and religious virtues (in that order) among the lower classes and to curtail the growing influence of the Catholic home-nursing organizations. On the other hand, they were appalled by the low standard of nursing in the urban poor law hospitals, which they set out to improve. Moreover, the liberal directors of the society thought nursing to be one of the few respectable activities in which ladies of comfortable backgrounds with a penchant for social work could engage themselves.[35] To this end the directors of the society aimed to train women of middle-class origin for home nursing. At first the number of suitable candidates was limited. Also, in order to obtain practical experience, these trainee home nurses had to be sent to work in precisely those urban poor law hospitals the directors deemed both medically and morally unsuitable. To solve these problems, the society founded in 1857 its own hospital, the Prinsengracht Ziekenhuis (Prinsengracht Hospital) in Amsterdam. Initially it did not differ in organization or medical care from the traditional urban institutions, but, in the eyes of the directors, the defects of poor law hospitals would be avoided by the respectable behavior of their own nurses. However, the hospital's charges were prohibitive for the poorer, private patients and poor law officials refused to pay for them. As a result, the number of patients remained low and the hospital failed to grow into a large, modern institution. The idea of hospital-based training for nurses was not realized and the society's nurses continued to devote their energy to home nursing. Only after 1903 did this hospital develop into a medical institution where hospital-based nurse training could take place.

As a secular model for the organization of home nursing, the Amsterdam Society for Sick Nursing had an enormous impact. Throughout the Netherlands it was the model for most of the home-nursing societies founded especially after 1870 and far into the twentieth century.[36] Their founders came from a variety of groups and organizations, including Red Cross departments, reformist physicians, and women's committees. All of these groups saw nursing as an acceptable profession for women; they tried to engage decent ladies, preferably from a middle-class background, who would be able, after limited training, to provide home nursing. For instance, the Haarlem Society for Sick Nursing, founded in 1871, gave their nurses a haphazard introduction to the principles of sick nursing in addition to free medical services and a small salary of $50 a year.[37]

Most societies employed a small number of nurses. In the 1870s, the Haarlem society employed only two nurses, and by 1900, at the height of its

popularity, no more than thirteen.[38] The education programs provided were short and subjects often randomly chosen. Furthermore, the nurses were often unable to attend the incidental lecture courses given by a local doctor, because they were on duty. In a few cases, nurses gained experience by working for a short period in a local poor law hospital, but more often this practice was not allowed and most therefore obtained experience in patients' homes. Sometimes nursing societies rented buildings where a few patients could be nursed, but these facilities rarely grew into modern hospitals.

The Emergence of Modern Nursing

Thus, at the beginning of the 1880s, two systems of nursing coexisted in the Netherlands. On the one hand, there were the public and communal hospitals that were intended for the poor and provided some medical care. Although a few nurses with at least minimal training were on duty in these hospitals, most of the nursing tasks were performed by untrained attendants. Furthermore, and more important, all these hospitals lacked training schools. On the other hand, there was an extensive network of societies and organizations of all denominations providing home nursing. Although the majority of these home-nursing societies gave at least some theoretical training, hospital apprenticeships were hard to negotiate.

Between 1880 and 1890, the first successful attempts were made to end this uneasy coexistence in Amsterdam. From the 1870s onward, the city witnessed a tremendous population increase; in thirty years the number of inhabitants almost doubled.[39] As a result, the pressure on the two most important traditional public hospitals of the city, the Binnen-Gasthuis (Inner Hospital) and the Buiten-Gasthuis (Outer Hospital) increased. Moreover, developments in medicine such as the introduction of antisepsis had convinced the progressive section of the local medical profession that modernization of the hospital system would have to include the introduction of the well-trained nurse. In 1883 the Amsterdam city council, supported by a few reformist physicians, started a revolution in the management of the Amsterdam public hospitals, which included employment of trained nurses. However, the problem the hospital boards faced was that such nurses were very hard to find.[40]

The first plans for a theoretical and practical training program for nurses were developed in Amsterdam in 1876 by some reformist doctors

who had founded the White Cross Organization.[41] Together with the liberal feminist Jeltje De Bosch Kemper (1836–1916), they planned to introduce nursing as a suitable and well-paid career for independent women. In 1879, a nursing school was founded to provide a one-year training program for nurses "within and without the public hospitals."[42] Its success, however, was seriously hampered by the difficulties of organizing practical experience for pupil nurses. In 1883 only seven nurses had been able to complete the White Cross training program.

Two people solved this deadlock, the newly appointed medical director of the Amsterdam Buiten-Gasthuis, Jacob van Deventer (1848–1916) and Johanna Paulina Reynvaan (1844–1920), a formidable organizer and later first matron of the Buiten-Gasthuis. Reynvaan, who came from a respectable Amsterdam family, had completed the one-year White Cross nursing program, but had only a few months' practical hospital experience because of the obstruction of the public hospital board.[43] Together, van Deventer and Reynvaan succeeded in reforming the Buiten-Gasthuis, founding the first hospital-based nurse training school, which in time came to supply the hospital with an able staff of trained nurses assisted by a growing body of pupil nurses.[44]

Although the Amsterdam reforms served as an acclaimed model, their example was not followed widely and was very often followed only halfheartedly. Some hospital boards were now prepared to employ nurses who had gained practical experience in home nursing. Others welcomed pupil nurses from home-nursing societies who were looking for an opportunity to improve their practical skills. Still others began to experiment with their own hospital-based training programs, adapting the curricula to their own requirements and needs.[45] The training programs, curricula, and examinations varied widely and ranged from a simple course in anatomy and physiology to complete two-year programs.

A crucial step in creating order out of the chaos was the founding in 1890 of the *Maandblad voor Ziekenverpleging* (Nursing Monthly) by, among others, Jeltje De Bosch Kemper and Johanna Reynvaan.[46] Kemper and Reynvaan had become close friends and in 1892 organized a major conference in Amsterdam which was attended by almost 200 delegates representing a range of societies and institutions that employed nurses or engaged in the organization of nurse training programs.[47] Striving for unity, the conference decided to found a new national organization, the Nederlandsche Bond voor Ziekenverpleging (Dutch Association for Sick Nursing), which, two years later, put forward a set of minimal requirements for hospital-based nurse training programs, with a trainee period of

three consecutive years in one hospital. Only those nurses who had passed their examination at one of the recognized hospitals could receive an official certificate. After 1905, due to an effective reorganization, the association succeeded in imposing its reforms on a steadily growing number of hospitals. Its system of nurse training finally became the model for government recognition in 1921.

Conclusion

There are some difficulties in comparing the development of nursing in the Netherlands to that of other countries. Though it seems that basic nursing concepts did not differ too much from country to country, variations occurred when people tried to apply these relatively similar concepts to the regulation and improvement of health care systems that were very different from each other in both structure and tradition.

Thus, due to the absence of such stimulating factors as war, colonial strife, and modern industrialization, hospital-based nursing took shape much later in the Netherlands than in other countries, such as England. In the 1880s industrial modernization and a complex series of medical reforms were responsible for the creation of a new hospital system. It spread across the country following the pattern of industrialization and urbanization, and by the 1920s the modern hospital was firmly entrenched in the Dutch medical landscape, almost eradicating the traditional public hospital. In a relatively short period of time, hospital nursing supplanted traditional home nursing. Instrumental in this process was the Dutch Association for Sick Nursing. In 1921, the Dutch government accepted as the basis of its regulations the models devised by the association. Thus, in the Nethlerlands, a uniform hospital-based training system took firm root almost simultaneously with the introduction of government recognition and a state examination system for the whole nursing profession. By the 1920s the modern Dutch nurse finally emerged.

NANNY WIEGMAN, RN, MA
Doctoral Candidate
Department of Medical History
Free University, Amsterdam
Van Der Boechorststraat 7
1081 BT Amsterdam
The Netherlands
Phone: 011 31 020-5482700

Acknowledgments

The research for this article was supported by a Wellcome Scholarship. I wish to thank the reviewers and Joan E. Lynaugh for their very helpful comments. I also want to thank Marijke Gijswijt-Hofstra, Claire Hengeveld, Annemarie de Knecht-Van Eekelen, and Hilary Marland for their critical suggestions and their assistance with the translation.

Notes

1. Morris J. Vogel, *The Invention of the Modern Hospital, Boston, 1870–1930* (Chicago: University of Chicago Press, 1985), 1–4.

2. See Susan McGann, *The Battle of the Nurses: A Study of Eight Women Who Influenced the Development of Professional Nursing, 1880–1930* (London: Scutari Press, 1992); and Celia Davies, "A Constant Casualty: Nurse Education in Britain and the USA to 1939," in *Rewriting Nursing History,* ed. Celia Davies (London: Croom Helm, 1980), 102–22.

3. Christopher J. Maggs, *The Origins of General Nursing* (London: Croom Helm, 1983), 9.

4. Literature in the English language on Dutch nursing is extremely scarce. But for some sharp insights, see *A History of Nursing from the Earliest Times to the Present Day with Special Reference to the Work of the Past Thirty Years,* ed. and in part written by Lavinia L. Dock (New York and London: G. P. Putnam's Sons, 1912), 55–74.

5. For a discussion of Dutch historiography, see Nanny Wiegman, "Zusters in Smetteloos Wit: een Blanco Bladzijde in de Nederlandse Geschiedschrijving?" *Tijdschrift voor de Geschiedenis der Geneeskunde, Natuurwetenschappen, Wiskunde en Techniek* 16, no. 2 (1993): 63–79 (hereafter cited as *GeWiNa*).

6. Anne Summers, *Angels and Citizens: British Women as Military Nurses, 1854–1914* (London: Routledge, 1988), 5–6.

7. J. C. Boogman, "The Netherlands in the European Scene, 1813–1913," in *Vaderlands Verleden in Veelvoud,* ed. G. A. M. Beekelaar (The Hague: Nijhoff, 1975), 481–96.

8. M. J. van Lieburg, "De Academisering van de Militair-Geneeskundige Opleiding in Nederland (1860–1880," "in *'s-Rijkskweekschool voor Militaire Geneeskundigen te Utrecht (1822–1865),* ed. D. de Moulin (Amsterdam: Rodopi, 1988), 91.

9. See G. M. Verspijck, *Het Nederlandsche Roode Kruis (1867–1967)* (Nijkerk: Callenbach, 1967), 69–76; A. R. J. Stumpel and M. J. van Lieburg, "Het Nederlandse Rode Kruis als Opleider van Verpleegsters, 1867–1897," *Spiegel Historiael* 19 (1984): 23–29; and M. J. van Lieburg, *Het Coolsingelziekenhuis te Rotterdam (1839–1900): De Ontwikkeling van een Stedelijk Ziekenhuis in de 19e Eeuw* (Amsterdam: Rodopi, 1986), 542–53.

10. Summers, 175–81.

11. See M. Kuitenbrouwer, *Nederland en de Opkomst van het Moderne Imperialisme* (Amsterdam: De Bataafsche Leeuw, 1985) 17–24; and H. L. Wesseling, "Dutch Historiography on European Expansion Since 1945," in *Reappraisals in Overseas History: Essays on Post-War Historiography About European Expansion,* ed. H. L. Wesseling and P. C. Emmer (Leiden: Leiden University Press, 1979), 138–39.

12. A. H. M. Kerkhoff, "The Organization of the Military and Civil Medical Service in the Nineteenth Century," in *Dutch Medicine in the Malay Archipelago, 1816–1942,* ed. A. M. Luyendijk-Elshout (Amsterdam: Rodopi, 1989), 9–24.

13. Martin Philip Bossenbroek, *Volk voor Indië: de Werving van Europese Militairen voor de Nederlandse Koloniale Dienst 1814–1909* (Amsterdam: Van Soeren, 1992).

14. Kerkhoff, 9.

15. See Vogel, 97–119; and Charles E. Rosenberg, *The Care of Strangers: The Rise of America's Hospital System* (New York: Basic Books, 1987), 100–103.

16. See J. A. de Jonge, *De Industrialisatie in Nederland tussen 1850 en 1914* (Nijmegen: SUN, 1976); R. T. Griffiths, *Industrial Retardation in the Netherlands, 1830–1850* (The Hague, 1979); and A. J. W. Camijn, *Een Eeuw vol Bedrijvigheid: De Industrialisatie van Nederland, 1814–1914* (Utrecht: Veen, 1987).

17. See De Jonge, 497–500; A. M. van der Woude, "Demografische Ontwikkeling van de Noordelijke Nederlanden 1500–1800," in *Algemene Geschiedenis der Nederlanden,* vol. 5 (Bussum: Unieboek, 1980), 134–39; and E. W. Hofstee, *Korte Demografische Geschiedenis van Nederland van 1800 tot Heden* (Bussum: Unieboek, 1981).

18. See P. B. A. Melief, *De Strijd om de Armenzorg in Nederland 1795–1854* (Groningen: Wolters, 1955); and P. A. C. Douwes, *Armenkerk: De Hervormde Diaconie te Rotterdam in de Negentiende Eeuw* (Schiedam: Interbook International, 1977).

19. See J. A. Verdoorn, *Het Gezondheidswezen te Amsterdam in de 19e Eeuw* (Nijmegen: SUN, 1981); C. A. Pekelharing, *Geschiedenis van de Vereenigde Gods- en Gasthuizen te Utrecht van 1817–1917* (Utrecht, 1921); M. J. van Lieburg, *'Een Nuttig en ten Sterkste Verlangd Wordend Hospitaal': De Geschiedenis van het Academisch Ziekenhuis Utrecht (1817–1992)* (Rotterdam: Erasmus Publishing, 1992); P. Kooji, *Groningen 1870–1914* (Assen: Van Gorcum, 1987); and J. Huizinga, *Memorabele Mensen en Momenten uit de Geschiedenis van de Intramurale Gezondheidszorg* (Lochem: De Tijdstroom, 1991), 148–49.

20. See Melief, 189–90; Douwes, 60–67; and J. A. A. Van Doorn, "De Strijd tegen Armoede en Werkeloosheid in Historisch Perspectief" in *Van Particuliere naar Openbare Zorg en terug?* ed. W. P. Blockmans and L. A. van der Valk (Amsterdam: NEHA, 1992), 1–30.

21. Nanny Wiegman, "Ziekenzorg in een Provinciehoofdstad (1833–1860): De Vroege Geschiedenis van het Stedelijk Ziekenhuis te Arnhem" (master's thesis, University of Nijmegen, 1990).

22. The most famous of these newly founded hospitals was the Burgerziekenhuis (Citizen's Hospital), which was founded in 1879 in Amsterdam. The hospital was meant for lower-middle-class patients and became a great success, especially after it acquired a new building in 1891. Cf. J. A. Groen, *Een Eeuw*

Burgerziekenhuis, 1879–1979 (Amsterdam, 1979); and J. A. Tours, "Het Burger-ziekenhuis te Amsterdam," in *Eigen Haard* (1889): 548–52.

23. M. J. van Lieburg, "De Verpleegkundige Literatuur in Nederland in de 19e Eeuw" *GeWiNa* 3, no. 3 (1980): 103.

24. See A. J. M. Alkemade, *Vrouwen XIX: Geschiedenis van Negentien Religieuze Congregaties, 1800–1850* ('s-Hertogenbosch: L. C. G. Malmberg, 1966); and José Eijt, "Zindelijkheid en Zuinigheid: De Voorbeeldfunctie van Vrouwelijke Religieuzen in de Ziekenverpleging gedurende de Negentiende Eeuw," *GeWiNa* 16, no. 2 (1993): 80–91.

25. Eijt, 88.

26. Gerard Pley, *Liefdewerk en Bejaardenzorg: Verkenningen in de Historie van de R. K. Stichting Verzorgings- en Verpleegtehuis Bernardus te Amsterdam, 1839–1989* (Amsterdam: R. K. Stichting Verzorgings- en Verpleegtehuis Bernardus, 1989).

27. See Rudolph Philips, *Gezondheidszorg in Limburg: Groei en Acceptatie van de Gezondheidsvoorzieningen, 1850–1940* (Assen: Van Gorcum, 1980), 86–87; M. J. van Lieburg, *Het Sint Franciscus Gasthuis te Rotterdam, 1892–1992* (Rotterdam: Erasmus Publishing, 1992), 40 43; and C. van Proosdij, *1891–1991: Honderd Jaar Hilversumse Ziekenhuishistorie* (Hilversum: Verloren, 1991), 17–30.

28. Recently the importance and quality of home and institutional nursing in the early nineteenth century in England has also been reevaluated. Cf. Carol Helmstadter, "Old Nurses and New: Nursing in the London Teaching Hospitals Before and After the Mid-Nineteenth-Century Reforms," *Nursing History Review* 1 (1993): 43–70. See also F. K. Prochaska, "Body and Soul: Bible Nurses and the Poor in Victorian London," *Historical Research: The Bulletin of the Institute of Historical Research* 60, no. 143 (October 1987), 336–48; Perry Williams, "Religion, Respectability and the Origins of the Modern Nurse," in *British Medicine in an Age of Reform,* ed. Roger French and Andrew Wear (London: Routledge, 1991), 231–55; and Anne Summers, "The Costs and Benefits of Caring: Nursing Charities, c.1830–c.1860," in *Medicine and Charity Before the Welfare State,* ed. Jonathan Barry and Colin Jones (London: Routledge, 1991), 133–48.

29. See L. J. Rogier, "Tachtig Jaar Katholieke Ziekenverpleging te Amsterdam," in *Aspecten van Caritas en Geneeskunde* (Amsterdam, 1958), 102–4; and Eijt, 88.

30. See G. N. M. Vis, *650 Jaar Ziekenzorg in Alkmaar 1341–1991: Hoofdstukken uit de Geschiedenis en Voorgeschiedenis van de Alkmaarse Zieken- en Gezondheidszorg* (Hilversum: Verloren, 1991), 130; and M. Briedé and H. F. M. Korthaus, *Zieken, Zorg en Zevenaar: De Geschiedenis van de Ziekeninrichtingen voor de Liemers* (Zevenaar: Stichting De Katholieke Ziekeninrichtingen voor de Liemers, 1992), 30–32.

31. A. B. R. du Croo de Vries, *Inventaris van het Archief van het Diakonessenhuis te Utrecht, 1844–1970* (Utrecht: Gemeentelijke Archiefdienst Utrecht, 1982), 7–11. It is still debatable whether the roots of the deaconess movement were German. When Theodor Fliedner visited the Netherlands in 1826, he came in contact with the work of deaconesses from the Doopsgezinde Church (Mennonite Church) and was very impressed by their organization. Cf. C. A. Drogendijk, *Het Protestants-Christelijk Ziekenhuis in Nederland* (Utrecht: Drukkerij Elinkwijk, 1975), 36.

32. The first matron of the institution, Miss A. H. Schwellengrebel, who was

matron for thirty years, was an extremely devout person, always trying to convert the patients first. Cf. *Her Diary* (1845), Archief Diakonessenhuis, inv. number, 212; and du Croo, 8.

33. Ten deaconess hospitals were founded between 1880 and 1900.

34. See J. A. Tours, "Iets over de Vereeniging voor Ziekenverpleging te Amsterdam en over Pleggzusters," in *Eigen Haard* (Amsterdam, 1889): 325–27; H. W. J. de Boer, *Prinsengracht Ziekenhuis: 25 Juli 1843–25 Juli 1983* (Amsterdam: Vereeniging voor Ziekenverpleging, 1983); and Herman W. J. de Boer and Gerard Pley, *"Grachtenzusters": Episoden uit Honderdvijftig Jaren Vereeniging voor Ziekenverpleging, sedert 1857 Gevestigd aan de Prinsengracht te Amsterdam* (Amsterdam, 1993).

35. De Boer, 17–18.

36. Cora Bakker-van der Kooij, "Mara. Pleegzuster zijn: Ontwikkelingen in de Ziekenverpleging en de Organisatiepogingen van Verpleegsters in Nederland, 1870–1920," *Tweede Jaarboek voor Vrouwengeschiedenis* (Nijmegen: SUN, 1981), 198.

37. "De Geschiedenis van de Haarlemse Vereniging voor Ziekenverpleging, 1871–1976," (Municipal Archive Haarlem, Inventaris Gemeente Archief), 77–91.

38. Ibid., 85.

39. In 1869 Amsterdam had 264,694 inhabitants. Its number increased to 510,853 in 1899. See Verdoorn, 28.

40. In 1883, during the reforms of the Amsterdam public hospitals, the hospital board had to introduce deaconnesses from Germany to reorganize the hospital nursing service. See *Vier Eeuwen Amsterdams Binnengasthuis: Drie Bijdragen over de Geschiedenis van een Gasthuis*, ed. D. de Moulin, I. H. Van Eeghen, and R. Meischke (Wormer: Inmerc B.V., 1981), 41–42.

41. The White Cross Organization was founded in 1875 to control and prevent infectious diseases.

42. See P. J. Barnouw, "Examens van het Witte Kruis," in *Maandblad voor Ziekenverpleging* 2, no. 3 (November 1891): 6; and B. S. H. Stieler and H. L. E. Van Den Berg, *Een Halve Eeuw Witte Kruis Arbeid, 1875–1925* (Amsterdam: M. J. Portielje, 1925).

43. Johanna W. A. Naber, *Het Leven en Werken van Jeltje de Bosch Kemper* (Haarlem: H. D. Tjeenk Willink & Zoon, 1918), 100.

44. Cf. *Maandblad voor Ziekenverpleging* 5, no. 11 (July 1895): 161–66.

45. For instance, the Rotterdamsch Sanatorium devised a two-year curriculum for in-service trainees, but also accepted paying pupils intent on a career in home nursing, who only attended theoretical classes and finished their nursing education with a four-week apprenticeship in the hospital each year. Cf. *Maandblad voor Ziekenverpleging* 2, no. 4 (December 1891): 12.

46. The *Maandblad* served as a clearing house for international news. The editorial board subscribed to foreign journals such as *Trained Nurse, Nursing Record,* and the German *Fortschritte der Krankenpflege.*

47. A full report of this congress was published in the nursing monthly *Maandblad voor Ziekenverpleging* 3, nos. 2 and 3 (October and November 1892): 33–83.

Linda Richards and Nursing in Japan, 1885–1890

MARY ELLEN DOONA
Boston College

Melinda Ann Judson Richards (1841–1930), nursing history's legendary first trained nurse, was directing nursing at the Boston City Hospital in 1879 when she "broke down in health." Colleagues cited overwork as the cause of her illness; her doctors diagnosed Richards's illness as "a moderately severe attack of neurasthenia."[1] Described as a want of nervous force analagous to anemia's want of blood, neurasthenia struck "brain workers" and people who had greater "sensibility" than most people.[2] Neurasthenia was a fashionable diagnosis for "mysterious nervous ailments, ranging from sick headaches, a becoming Victorian delicacy, to screaming hysteria and psychosis."[3] Richards was "critically ill for many weeks and only regained her health by slow and prolonged recovery" at the McLean Hospital in Somerville, Massachusetts, where she was treated with a modified version of the "enforced rest treatment" then in vogue.[4] During this time she was also treated for "pulmonary and pelvic disease." Richards herself named her illnesses "lung and nervous trouble."[5]

Very little information of Richards's inner life survives, but the little that does is of this time. She was thirty-eight years old when the illness began and forty when she returned to work. She was already past the age her sister (thirty-two) and father (thirty-six) had been when they died, and nearing the age (forty-two) at which her mother had died of consumption when Richards was only thirteen years old. Her mother's illness and death had prompted in Richards a spiritual awakening, and she joined the Baptist Church. Twenty-two years later, as she recuperated from her own illness, Richards underwent another religious renewal. She confessed, "I think I have been renewed by the Holy Spirit — because I love the word of God as

Nursing History Review 4 (1996): 99–128. Copyright © 1996 by The American Association for the History of Nursing.

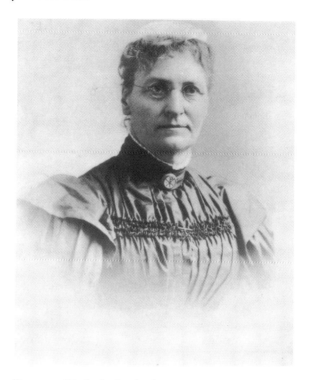

Figure 1. Linda Richards during her missionary work with the ABCFM. (By permission of Houghton Library, Harvard University, and United Church Board for World Ministries)

once I did not. I love the Children of God . . . I love prayer [and] I take pleasure in the law of God."[6]

Richards's religious rebirth coincided with a militant Christianity in the United States that saw itself divinely ordained to export to the world its Protestant Christianity in time for the resurrection expected at the millennium. Though women missionaries exceeded the number of men in missionary work, they exercised none of the authority, reflecting the general pattern of life in the nineteenth century. But single women especially found missionary work a socially sanctioned arena of activity and freedom. Under the fostering care of the Church, Protestant women found definition beyond husband and children as they followed their own will and conscience.[7] Richards became a special instance of this nineteenth-century Protestant feminism.

"Our Little Torch" — The Women's Board of Missions

Richards had wanted to be a missionary since she had been a child listening to returned missionaries tell of their work.[8] The "Ann Judson" part of her name — given to her by her father — was a constant reminder of the first single woman missionary, Ann Hasselton Judson (1789–1826).[9] These childhood memories reawakened when Richards heard of the need for a nurse to set up a training school in Kyoto. She eagerly offered her services to John C. Berry, a doctor who had been with the Japanese mission since 1872. Berry represented N. G. Clark, the secretary of the American Board of Commissioners of Foreign Missions (ABCFM), which had helped found a missionary school in Kyoto called the *DoShisha* (precursor to DoShisha University). Berry had not met Richards, but from her reputation judged her to be a "woman of rare ability, thoroughly qualified in her profession and of mature Christian character."[10] Clarke responded, "We are all more and more impressed with her as the right woman for the right place, and one who will work pleasantly and genially with all."[11] And like many women of her time Richards romanticized the position and envisioned "hardship, suffering and peril" as she imagined herself a missionary "leading souls to Christ."[12]

RICHARDS JOINS THE PROTESTANT FEMINISTS

Richards joined the parade of single women missionaries which had begun in 1861 with one woman and would by 1909 total 4,710.[13] Her predecessors and contemporaries were teachers determined to elevate the status of women by educating and at the same time converting them to Christianity. Richards's training school would educate these women for nursing and then they would carry the Christian message to their patients. The Women's Board of Missions (WBM), which underwrote the expenses of a training school and hospital, reflected women of the nineteenth century and their growing commitment to shape the world in which they lived. The WBM had decided that "their own peculiar duty [was] towards their benighted sisters in heathen lands," and persuaded other women that it was their obligation to support such efforts. They visualized 300,000,000 "benighted sisters" in Asia alone "waiting for the blessing of the gospel" and receiving at "the hands of their more favored sisters the bread of life, [as] the light of the gospel [was] . . . borne by gentle hands into their darkened homes."[14] More important, following the precepts of Mary Lyons (1797–1849), the founder of Mt. Holyoke Female Seminary, the WBM imagined single women missionaries not as helpmates to men but as real missionaries serv-

ing as chaplains and spiritual advisors.[15] Safely nestled in Boston's Beacon Hill parlors, this determined group of women sent missionaries to exotic places and imagined ancient cultures transformed into their own New England image.

A rock-hard Yankee realism shaped their idealism. In 1885, the year Linda Richards decided to be a missionary, the ABCFM found itself in the awkward position of having to ask the WBM to extend its support to the wives of missionaries. The sense of autonomy felt by the WBM can be seen in their refusal of the male clerics' request for $25,000. Though the women graciously acknowledged the "excellency of the ladies" and their sisterhood with them, the WBM kept its finances focused on the single woman missionary. Interestingly, they prefaced this refusal by reading Romans 16, in which St. Paul speaks of Phoebe, a deaconess in the early church.[16] Earlier that year at the February meeting, they pledged $3,000 for a home for young ladies in Kyoto and $5,000 for the training school for nurses. They designated $83,000 more for other projects for a one-year total expenditure of $102,080 in 1989 dollars.[17]

KUDOS AND CONSTRAINTS

At their August 1885 meeting, the women read the testimonials written on behalf of Richards. A personal reference praised Richards as a devoted Christian woman and "one of my most helpful friends."[18] Mary Prescott of Foxboro, Massachusetts, who had known Richards for twenty years, wrote of her as being self-sacrificing, devoted, remarkably cheerful, and hopeful. Moreover, she had "great energy and persistence in carrying out her plans once begun."[19] Edward Cowles, Richards's medical colleague at Boston City Hospital, wrote from his new post as superintendent at the McLean Hospital saying, "If I were engaged in the management of such a work, I would choose her first of all the women I know."[20] His successor at Boston City Hospital, George Rowe, who had told Richards of the Japanese mission, added, "My admiration for the woman, her ability, training, Christian character and strong personal regard for her leads me to speak of her in the highest praise. . . . There is no one who is her equal [in] intellectual and executive ability, energy, practical experience, commonsense [sic] and sound judgment. She has eminently excelled in her work at the hospital and we should be very sorry to have her go from us." Rowe also mentioned that Richards was a very good judge of character.[21]

Later Rowe regretted this recommendation because he wanted Richards to stay at Boston City Hospital. He tried to discredit her appropri-

ateness as a missionary on the grounds of her past illness. A determined Richards enlisted the aid of her medical colleagues in her contest with the imperious Rowe.[22] Berry wrote his superiors, "She is respected deeply and much honored by those among whom she moves in her daily life and many a weaker woman would have been turned from her purpose by the arguments . . . of those who would keep her where she now is. . . . It was evident that their wish that she should not go preceded their opinion that she could not go. . . . I judge her to be a rare prize — such a one as it would be hard to find anywhere else in the country." Berry was less obvious than Rowe in his paternalistic style, but he, too, was a man of his times, and saw Richards as his helpmate and assistant.[23]

When the WBM voted on 31 August 1885 to adopt Richards for the training school in Kyoto, Japan, Richards was once again within a female network of support that she had enjoyed as a student at the feminist showplace, the New England Hospital for Women and Children, and as a graduate nurse at the Bellevue Hospital and the Boston Training School. The WBM would arrange for suitable company, pay her passage to Japan, and provide her with a suitable residence and the facilities for learning the Japanese language. The WBM would also meet her necessary expenses and pay her $650, a reduction in her usual salary but the same as other single women missionaries, while she was "in the field."[24] In return, Richards was expected to remain in Japan for five years, provide an annual report, and correspond with the WBM, notifying it of her condition and the progress of the work done under her charge. Excerpts from these letters would be published in the WBM's journal, *Light and Life*. Richards agreed to these terms and wrote, "I hope I may be able in the strength of Him who is always able and willing to help us, to do the work you have so kindly appointed me to — and to do it faithfully and well."[25]

After a "God-speed meeting," Richards said good-bye to her Boston friends. Now freed from all encumbrances, Richards turned her back on the tenets of modern nursing which she had followed for twelve years. With her decision to become a missionary nurse, she was returning to pre-Crimean War nursing, when nursing was done by the church. Then, nursing was a moral matter; church women cared for the body as the means by which they gained access to the soul of their patients. After the Crimean War (1854–56), nursing became secularized; any woman could nurse, and, more important, nursing now focused on the prevention and cure of disease, not the salvation of souls. Richards's new identity as a missionary nurse was grounded in the old idea of nursing.[26]

Opportunity for Wide Influence

Richards had emerged from the dark wood of her illness, and midway on her journey through life, she struck out on this new path. She left Boston on 14 December 1885. During her trip across America she visited old friends and spent the Christmas holiday with a former colleague in Los Angeles. When her steamer arrived in Honolulu, a missionary, Mr. Damon, sent to the boat for any missionaries, and found only Richards. He, his wife, and his mother then took Richards on a seven-hour tour about the town and made calls on other missionary families. These visits and a dinner with the family of Rev. Mr. Merritt, the president of Oahu College, validated Richards's new identity as a missionary. Two more weeks on board the steamer brought Richards to Japan. At midnight on 24 January 1886, the ship sailed into Kobe harbor.[27]

The next day she mailed her letters and stopped at a silk shop to buy a birthday gift for her sister before traveling by ricksha to the Bible house. She protested that she did not like to "see men used as horses," but this would be her mode of transportation throughout her time in Japan.[28] Berry came from Kyoto to Kobe to welcome her and to accompany her on the last leg of her journey. After six weeks of traveling from Boston to Japan, Richards arrived on 27 January 1886 in the cradle and stronghold of Buddhism and exclaimed, "At last I am in Kioto!"[29]

Richards was eager to begin her work, but on her arrival she found that the DoShisha had not purchased the land on which the training school and hospital were to be built. The training school, like the DoShisha itself, was a joint operation, with the Japanese supplying the land and buildings and the ABCFM supporting the teachers, the apparatus of the school, and the work itself. Richards's first day in Kyoto was spent touring the proposed sites with Berry and a Japanese professor. She was delighted to hear that there was much interest in the training school and plenty of prospective students.

ARRIVAL AND DEPARTURE

The missionaries welcomed Richards into their American village, which was completely devoid of the Japanese culture surrounding it. Although Richards thought the missionaries were as happy a people as she had ever seen, her first task suggested that not all was happiness in the American compound. The melancholy wife of one of the missionaries had become seriously depressed following the delivery of her baby. Her depression failed to respond to supportive treatment — cod liver oil, iron, and maltine.

Worse, the depression was deepening and the woman's thinking became delusional. Berry, who cared for the missionary personnel as well as the Japanese, ordered a complete change of climate. Richards cordially accepted the duty, saying, "As I was useless now, it was thought best for me to go to Shanghai with her for a time. Her husband goes too, of course, but some of the missionaries would have had to go and so they asked me, giving me liberty to decide. There will be little to be done for [the woman] by way of nursing, still she needs some one."[30]

Richards was happy to help out the mission and hoped that while she cared for the depressed woman in China, she could learn Japanese, but there was little leisure to devote to mastering Japanese during the next three months. When she and the missionary wife returned to Japan, the woman was physically improved, but ominously, the delusion that she had committed an unpardonable sin remained unchanged. Berry then decided the woman and her family should leave Japan for the more stimulating environment of California. This relieved Richards of her duty but proved disastrous for the depressed woman. On the second day of her voyage west, somewhere between Kobe and Yokohama, she slipped away from her caretakers and plunged into the sea to her death.[31]

The tragic loss of the young mother and the mix-up about the training school foreshadowed events to come. The reality of caring for the depressed American fell far short of Richards's dream of peril as she converted heathen women. The mission, however, was grateful for her services and the ABCFM praised Richards for increasing the moral strength and courage of the women missionaries just by being there with them.[32] In the meantime, mission life continued and Richards attended socials and prayer meetings, but she felt useless as she saw everyone but herself hard at work. Still, she was very happy, she assured the ABCFM.

In August, Richards went to Hiyeison mountain with the other missionaries for a combination of vacation and mission meeting. From there she wrote to friends in Boston of her eager pursuit of Japanese with the help of her teacher and a dictionary. She enjoyed the Japanese people as far as she knew them, and described them as "patient and cheerful — and though they are slow they are faithful." Keeping her focus on the training school, she added, "I think they will make good nurses."[33] Richards was typical of the new missionary that seasoned workers pleaded with the home office *not* to send to Japan. They wanted each missionary to have spent three years studying the language and becoming acquainted with the Japanese people before taking up any responsible work. Still, these early months helped

Richards become acclimated to Japan, though in the five years she spent there she never became acculturated.

THE CAMPAIGN FOR THE TRAINING SCHOOL

Then Nee-Sima, the founder and president of the DoShisha, published his campaign for the nurses' training school in twenty of the leading Japanese college periodicals. After introducing the history of modern nursing, Richards's leadership in the United States, and the proposed training school, the pamphlet listed the requirements of applicants. They should be between thirty and forty years of age, in sound health, and of good character. Like their counterparts in the United States, applicants were expected to be sober, honest, truthful, trustworthy, punctual, quiet, orderly, cleanly, patient, kind, and cheerful. They had to be quick and careful in observation and able to read the Scriptures intelligently.

The course of study also reflected American training schools. It was eighteen months or more in length, and work in the wards of the hospital and practical work in district nursing among the city's sick poor was combined with theory classes from textbooks in nursing, anatomy, physiology, and hygiene. Pupils would be taught to be loyal to the physician, increase the confidence of the patients in their doctors, and in every possible way cooperate with them. Lessons in the Scriptures were also required. At the successful completion of the course, graduates would be given a diploma.

Civil authorities took strong exception to the requirement that all candidates for admission were required to be able to read the Scriptures. This was proof enough for them that the school was being founded for sectarian purposes and that the Japanese were being asked to "abandon the religion of [their] fathers to support an alien faith."[34] Public funds should not be used for a religious school, they argued. This reasoning was countered by those who said they would support any enterprise because it *contained* such a clause. If Christianity was the source of the ten-year-old DoShisha's strength, they said, the more of the Bible and Christianity that Japanese institutions could have, the better. This was especially so in the training school because the work of nursing was "too dirty and difficult to be done by anyone unless they [*sic*] are helped by something more than ordinary strength."[35] Still another problem was that the head of the school was both a foreigner and a woman.

In the midst of these church-state, native-foreigner arguments, on 21 May 1886, cholera broke out in the city. Richards offered her services but the civil authorities refused them, fearing that she would be exposed to the

infection. Her gesture was a public relations success of the first magnitude. The Japanese proclaimed her generous offer and then stressed the urgent need for a training school because in Japan "skilled nursing [is] almost unknown."[36]

Nee-Sima, who had a profound belief in the power of education to transform Japanese civilization, continued his campaign, saying, "We do not establish this institution in order merely to spread Christianity, rather we receive courage from Christianity to enable us to do this work for humanity. Our friends in America, too, do not give us help merely to spread Christianity in Japan though this of course is remembered in establishing a work: rather, they do this for suffering humanity because strength of heart and purpose which Christian truth has developed in their hearts seeks this and every . . . opportunity for helpful activity."[37] By August 1886, Nee-Sima had enough money to purchase land for the complex. The campaign was a success, though, to be sure, the opposition was not completely dissolved, as events five years later would reveal. A kind of real estate speculation developed as each affordable piece of land suddenly became more expensive once the DoShisha selected it. One owner had "gone up so much in his price," wrote Richards, "that now it does not look as though there was much prospect of getting this lot." At the same time, the ABCFM had to reduce its expenditures in Japan. The higher cost of real estate and reduced support from Boston slowed even more the plans for the training school. Richards was vexed with the tempo of missionary work, finding it far slower than nursing in the United States. "It requires a good deal of patience for an energetic New England woman to get on comfortably here," she wrote. "I must say I have a task before me to learn to be patient, but I mean to do it."[38]

Planting an Institution

In the fall of 1886, Richards accepted the first class of five students, using the house of her unfortunate American patient as hospital, pharmacy, nurses' home, classroom, and her own home. She complained that she was never able to have privacy or the necessary change from work: "While I would not mind living in the same home I feel that one would wear out sooner by so doing. My hours with the Japanese must be many during the day. From early morning till late at night and I feel that to be where they could not come to me by just knocking at the door would be a more sure

way of getting rest when off duty. All tired people complain of the strain of continually listening to the language. This I must hear from morning till night." Richards worried about her own health, adding, "So far I am strong and well — and I do want to work years in Japan and I trust I may."[39] Unlike the other single women missionaries, the teachers, Richards could not retreat from her work to the comforts of a home. Nor did she have a colleague with whom to share a missionary life. In the beginning, Richards had few respites from this loneliness. Women such as Fannie Gardner (1849–1930) lived with Richards as they underwent medical treatment, and provided her with much needed companionship. Once recovered, they returned to their own missionary work and Richards was alone again with nurses and patients.

EVANGELIZING: A GRAND WORK

Richards stressed her need for an associate and reminded the WBM that its fundamental objective in founding the training school was to evangelize Japanese women. She wanted an associate who would spend some time each day doing evangelical work among the sick in the hospital. This would be still another new role for single women missionaries, because up to that time, they had been teachers. Married ladies did all they could, said Richards, and she emphasized the distinction between single and married women in the mission. "No lady with a family and its cares and work," wrote Richards, "can do what a single lady with all her time to work among the people can do."[40]

Richards worried about all the lost opportunities to preach to patients during the crisis of illness when they could be "more easily reached."[41] She also worried that the lessons patients heard about Christianity at the hospital were often forgotten when they returned home. Converting Japanese women from Buddhism to Christianity was an enormous task and Richards sought recruits, saying that "women are wanted in this country and the lady who wished to come as nurse might do a grand work as a general missionary among women." She looked to the day when a home large enough for two people would be built and someone would come to Japan to do the evangelistic work in the hospital. Then the training school would be firmly established and a "real help in spreading the knowledge of the gospel" in Japan.[42]

Superintending the training school was such an all-consuming work that Richards had very little leisure and less freedom to go beyond the confines of the hospital and training school. She rose in the morning at six o'clock and worked till ten-thirty or eleven at night, but even then she went

to bed feeling that she had left much undone.[43] She had few stretches of free time. Even letter writing had "to be picked up and put down much as I pick up and put down my knitting work."[44] Richards was as restricted by the training school and hospital as the wives of missionaries were by their husbands and children.

Throughout this time, other missionaries wrote to Boston on behalf of Richards. Berry reminded the home office of Richards's need for a "house . . . not a room in a dormitory with students." In December, he declared that "Miss Richards is too valuable a person not to provide for with the greatest care. She is wholly self-forgetful, however, and would be content, if there was no help for it, in a native hovel." He remarked, too, that Miss Richards was "cooking over a brazier surrounded by the sick."[45] Under such pressure, the WBM allocated $2,000 on 18 April 1887 for Richards's home, "a place to [her]self— [her]castle free from all intruders."[46]

Meanwhile, Richards taught her students in Berry's medical clinic and the makeshift hospital where, as she told her friends in Boston, "We have mostly lung cases [and] . . . eye cases. Eyes and lungs seem to be weak points here." Though this was ordinary and perhaps boring nursing for Richards, it was not so for its recipients. One old lady who had been totally blind for a long time was amazed when she could see the doctor after cataract surgery. The woman was so happy she could not eat. Still, Richards felt she was doing "very little."[47]

Richards was pleased with her first class of Japanese pupil nurses. She reported,

> The five nurses are doing well; some of them remarkably well. The work is hard, and we have all worked hard this winter, and the nurses have been most uncomplaining. Any new work is hard and taking care of people in a house not convenient for well people is surely not easy work. But we hope that before many months we will be in a little Hospital. And we could fill quite a large hospital had we had one to fill. We are constantly saying "no room." Some of our people have become much interested in Christianity and have gone to their homes saying they would study it carefully. And we do feel that the work done here is doing good to souls as well as to bodies. The nurses here are all Christian women and each one tries to lead others to Christ.[48]

The construction of the training school and hospital buildings began during the spring of 1887. In the midst of this, Richards was asked to share her little home in the hospital with a missionary woman who had sustained a concussion subsequent to a fall from a ricksha. After a six-week period of bed rest, she slowly recovered from the fall, but then was diagnosed with "ovarian irritation." At times, especially during her menses, she suffered

"hysterical convulsions" and was "quite out of her mind." Her physician, Sara Craig Buckley, feared brain softening. Richards looked after the patient and oversaw her treatment with sedatives, tonics, galvanism, and scheduled amounts of exercise and rest each day. This was probably similar to the treatment she herself had received during her own illness prior to coming to Japan. As Richards got to know the woman and her past history, she concluded correctly that the woman had probably been nervous for years before she came to Japan.[49] Buckley's summary of the case provides a window on late-nineteenth-century care.

> Miss Richards was constantly watching her and with a nurse's assistance [the patient] was never left alone so she would not overdo in any way. The least exertion on her part would excite her and she would suffer insomnia and would take several days to recover. She did nicely [for four weeks] and again she was worse, this time having severe meningitis symptoms followed by catalepsy and hysterical insanity. She is constantly growing worse. . . . [We] decided to send her home at once, so that she might be under the care of a specialist in nervous diseases, for we feel if anything is done, it must be done at once. As you well know the climate in Japan is very depressing for all nervous diseases. . . . [A]ll kinds of nervous troubles that have remained have become worse.[50]

Richards and a Japanese girl accompanied the woman "who ha[d] to be carefully watched, her mind not being right at all times and one cannot take care of her on such a journey." The doctor on the steamer echoed the general feeling among the missionaries that the woman should not have been sent out. "She is not a girl who should leave her friends," said the steamer doctor. He predicted correctly that she would regain her health soon after she reached home.[51] By the next year, Richards had gained more experience with the kind of person not suited for missionary life. "The longer I am in Japan," she said, "the more I am convinced that nervous people and particularly those who are hysterically inclined should never come here and I feel very strongly that many can do good work at home who could not do good work here."[52] It was with this new-found perspective that Richards told Buckley and the WBM, "When I am in a condition to necessitate some member of the mission (who can work for the Japanese) leaving her work to take care of me, I am to be sent home. I came here to work and when I cannot work and must be taken care of I do not want to weaken the Mission by having some one take care of me. So when I can no longer work, you will see me home."[53]

While in Boston, Richards dropped in on the WBM. The secretary

tersely summarized, "Miss R[ichards] was present and at this point in the meeting occupied considerable time in a very interesting report of her work."[54] Unknown is whether Richards unloaded her heart or advised the ladies of the WBM about the problems of women in the Japanese mission. Still, her own commitment to missionary life remained firm and after a few weeks she returned to Kyoto.

A HOME OF HER OWN

On 5 November 1887, Richards moved into the home promised her when she signed up with the mission. She was delighted with her new house, and thanked the ladies of the WBM effusively, remarking that she had not realized how uncomfortable she had been until she moved into a home of her own. Buckley and her husband lived with Richards while they waited for their own house to be finished. Two years after her arrival, Richards not only had a house, she finally lived in a home with people whose company she enjoyed.[55]

Ten days later the entire training school complex was finished. Along with Richards's home, there were hospital buildings and a two-story training school building. Five hundred and fifty prominent Japanese came to the dedication, and over 3,000 people — physicians and health and government officers — inspected the buildings. Following the tour, services were held in the DoShisha chapel, after which there was a reception. With the completion of the hospital/training school complex, all that Richards needed now was an associate.

Richards's fervor for evangelizing the Japanese continued unabated. She was astonished at the Japanese "craze for English and foreign ways."[56] Only 34 years had passed since the opening of Japan after 200 years of self-imposed isolation. Since than, Japan had been transformed by transportation, telegraph, and technology. Richards reported that the Japanese were "reaching after western civilization and knowledge, but what they need is Christianity." As ethnocentric as the rest of the mission, Richards seemed oblivious to the Buddhist religion except as an enemy of "the truth." She visited the temples that dotted the hillsides of Kyoto, but was aghast at the thousands going to worship at them and overwhelmed at how much more work needed to be done to convert the Japanese from Buddhism to Christianity.[57] But she never asked about Buddhism nor why the Japanese were so faithful.

The enormous task of conversion weighed on her and added to the burden of the nursing work. Richards often complained of her fatigue.

"But," she said, "when one has to be dressmaker to the nurses besides all the other things which at home other people do, it may not be wondered at that one tires out."[58] Berry, who had been with the mission for more than fifteen years and seemed more acclimated to the missionary pace, thought Richards got "very nervous over the many little cares and annoyances incident to her position (such as keeping the nurses straight and caring for the wards) and grows tired under it."[59] Berry's own work with patients was aided by Richards's twenty-four-hour-a-day oversight of the hospital, but Richards had no one to help her. She found that student nurses often did not carry out her orders, though to be fair to the students, these orders were often given through an interpreter and may have been misunderstood. She constantly had to check on their work, and under this relentless burden of responsibility, Richards grew querulous. As one of the missionaries told Richards, she "was fast becoming old in Japan. [A]nd so I am," Richards realized.[60]

Although increasingly fatigued by the task of educating students, Richards basked in the "glorious work" of evangelization. She attended the twice-weekly prayer meeting in the nurses' home, the weekly prayer meeting at the DoShisha church, morning prayers for all employees of the hospital, and evening prayers in each patient's room. Richards and Buckley also lectured each week to the Women's Improvement Society. In addition to all this, Richards visited daily a sick woman who lived three miles from the hospital. After lecturing five hours a day in the school and overseeing patient care in the hospital, Richards wrote letters to churches who had sent money to the school. Buckley praised Richards's "work of love. Of course, the Hospital could not run without her, both on account of her Hospital training and fine executive abilities." Later she added, "I think Providence surely sent [Richards] to us and I value the privilege of having her with us more and more."[61]

In November Buckley stressed that Richards needed "some one very much to assist her and relieve her when she is feeling poorly." She testified that "everyone, both foreign and Japanese, loves her and so she is able to exert a wide influence in all."[62] Her missionary colleagues were increasingly aware of the value of the training school. Indeed, Berry reported that the school was "regarded with growing favor among the people and the hospital work is exerting a wide influence for good."[63] The Christian message the missionaries were trying to convey, often through an interpreter who may have missed the nuances in the message, was more accurately conveyed in the care given by Richards and her pupils. Richards felt compelled to do

more. "I am strong," said Richards ever mindful of her health, "but have not strength for all, if I had the time — nor can I do both well."[64]

Flora Denton, a teacher who arrived in Kyoto in 1888 and would stay there the rest of her life, came to live with Richards once the Buckleys moved into their own house. She, too, was anxious for Richards and reported that she worked "very very hard." She was more aware than Berry of how unremitting Richards's work was. When Denton saw that even Richards's rest time was used helping the nurses with their uniforms, she tried to persuade the WBM to send out a sewing machine. When the machine was not forthcoming, Denton told the WBM to charge it to her own salary if no other source was available.[65] Neither Richards nor Denton sought the simpler solution of allowing the Japanese students to wear their own native garb. Still, Denton was more forthright than either Richards or Buckley when she wrote to the WBM. She tried to translate women's numbers in the mission into power to shape policy. She reminded the WBM that single missionary women were not to be ignored. She asked them to please remember that "we constitute a family [and] our address is Doshisha Hospital." Furthermore, she directed the WBM that when they made out their lists, they should not overlook "this family." Though this family composed of single women missionaries was certainly not the ideal Protestant family of male authority and female subordination, nonetheless they were a family, said Denton, and deserved all the favors at least that are shown to other families.[66] But Denton's demand did not change the fact that though the women far outnumbered the men, the mission men exercised the authority.[67]

Denton was just as forthright in her assessment of Richards. She enjoyed living with her and reported, "It is a very great privilege to be allowed to live with Miss Richards. She is a most successful worker and she has none of the little whims and cranks that some time make very lovely Christians, very disagreeable people. She has been the greatest help to me in every way. The work . . . in this school is very grand. Miss Richards works without a thought to herself."[68]

Wanted: A Noble Woman As an Associate

In June 1888, four nurses, the first graduates of the DoShisha Training School for Nurses, received their nursing diplomas. The second class of seven had completed their first year, and the third would enter that fall.

Although she now had a woman living with her, Richards still had 100 percent of the burden of the training school. So heavy was this responsibility that Richards spent her vacation in Maiko trying to recover her health and to replenish her energy for the fall term. She was enormously disappointed, saying that she had had "two of the hardest years (as far as work goes) here in Kyoto that I ever had in my life and it ha[d] not been as successful as the amount of work would indicate to one outside."[69]

Looking back on that summer from the vantage point of October, Richards recalled leaving the hospital in August "feeling more nearly sick than [she had] ever done in the year before. . . . [She] spent more than half the time in bed." Even though she came near having pneumonia, she was unable to rest because there was "no one to do the work." Her fatigue was exacerbated by her fear of lung disease, a fear grounded in the reality of her family's history of consumption. But the work took priority over her health and Richards worked from her bed, undermining any recovery of strength and health.[70]

Buckley reported that Richards's resistance to infection was lowered because of exhaustion and overwork and then gave the course of the infection in the preantibiotic nineteenth century. When Richards left for vacation in Maiko, she was "weak and prostrated. Before leaving she had some pain in her left ear, after reaching there the inflammation of the middle ear extended and after several days of severe pain it broke. So soon as this was better the other ear also passed through the same process, and then it returned again to the left ear which again broke. Tonsillitis followed, and now that her throat is better the disease has extended to her lungs, and she is now weak and has been losing flesh, while her cough troubles her very much. I feel sure this has all been excited by overwork, and the prostration that followed it."[71] At this point, Richards seriously considered returning to the United States, but Denton and Buckley persuaded her to remain in Japan.

A NURSE, NOT AN EVANGELIST

Realizing that she would not be getting a single woman missionary as an associate, Richards began to ask for a trained nurse. Once that nurse was acclimated to Japan, she could take over much of the nursing work. Then, thought Richards, she herself would be free to rest and manage the evangelical work among the Japanese women. Her missionary colleagues "on the ground" agreed to this proposition. Richards did not leave the search for a nurse only to the missionary boards. She wrote to friends in the

United States trying to persuade them to come to Japan, or if they could not come themselves to recommend someone who would. Few had the freedom to do so, even had they the inclination. Richards despaired that any help could be found and "no one seems to offer."[72]

Richards continued to write to the WBM and asked for a "noble woman." She hoped for the right nurse, a devoted Christian woman, who would adapt to missionary nursing. She should be someone "who could be happy without the conveniences of a Boston hospital" and who would realize before she came that she was not "coming into sun shine only." [Emphasis in original.][73] At last, Boston wrote that Miss Ida V. Smith, of Wichendon, Massachusetts, an 1883 graduate of Mary Lyons' Mount Holyoke Female Seminary and an 1888 graduate of the Connecticut Training School, was on her way.[74] "The hope of seeing Miss Smith," wrote the elated Richards, "has restored me a great deal." She continued in happy anticipation, saying, "I shall go to Kobe to meet her and bring her back to her new home and I shall try very hard to make her happy."[75] Richards promised that Smith would get a "very warm welcome" into the happy home she shared with Denton.[76] Relief and gratitude quickly gave way to anxiety about how Smith would perceive the training school. There were fewer applicants than expected, due in part to the competition from a school in Tokyo. Moreover, these applicants were less promising than their predecessors. Richards was concerned that Smith would find them slow and get discouraged, and then confessed she herself had been discouraged many times. Smith arrived in Kyoto on Christmas Eve 1888. She was no Christmas gift by any stretch of the imagination; Smith would prove to be a lethal mix of inexperience and overconfidence. Berry worried about the "healthy, pleasant and very promising lady" because she was a little homesick and somewhat disappointed when she first arrived. Smith would not be able to do much of the work, but whether this was because of Smith's inexperience — she had only graduated from training school that year — or newness to Japan, Berry did not say. He was confident, however, that within six months "everything will, I think, be all right."[77]

Berry had explicitly directed the ABCFM to select an appropriate associate for Richards. He asked the ABCFM to be very careful to choose a person who would be thoroughly loyal to Richards and would be willing to take a second place for some time. Then, after years of experience she would be able to take full charge when Miss Richards needed rest. "Inexperience will not work harm at first," thought Berry, "for she can learn from Miss Richards and gain a rich experience from day to day."[78]

Smith would soon enough show how wrong Berry was, but during her first days in Kyoto, she wrote delightedly of her new post:

> If you could see Miss Richards surrounded by her class of women all eagerly intent upon her words, she in as much earnest as any [of them] more so to make her meaning clear to them, you would not wonder that I am almost desperately impatient to gain enough of the language to be at work, too. . . . Those of you who know Miss Richards' personality I know feel like congratulating me for being with one so lovely in every way — full of Christian grace and patience, instead of allowing me to feel my utter hopelessness, she has arranged for me little duties, already in connection with my study — the things of comparatively little importance to give me the feeling of doing something in the work.[79]

Smith enthused that "Dr Berry has been kindness itself to me in these first trying days when one feels so helpless and had it not been for him I should have been heartsick and discouraged many times."[80]

Unlike Berry and Smith, Richards was silent. Some of the silence might be attributed to a pressing problem that threatened the integrity of the school. The wife of one of the missionaries refused a nurse that Richards sent to be with her during her confinement and demanded another. Berry overrode Richards's decision, setting the precedent for undermining her authority, and the woman got the nurse she wished for. Then she refused to pay the nurse's fee until the mission forced her to do so. The woman had had a long history of difficulties in the mission, first as a single woman missionary and then as the wife of a missionary. Earlier in her missionary career as a teacher, she had become very nervous and thin. Berry had tried to block her return to Japan after a period of rest and recovery in the United States, but the women in the mission pleaded her cause. Several years later when she was to deliver her baby, she had so alienated these and other women that no women in the mission were willing to help her. Richards became the target of this woman's vengeance. Richards would be vindicated, but not until the woman's demands had become so extravagant that the entire family was sent home, in spite of the husband's reputation as one of the DoShisha's most outstanding professors. By that time the wife had caused a great deal of misfortune, as events to come would bear out.

This was a difficult problem to be sure, but it does not completely explain Richards's silence. Three months passed and then Richards reported tersely that Miss Smith had arrived safely and was doing all she could in studying the language. The WBM should have suspected that something was amiss and Richards should have been more forthright. But

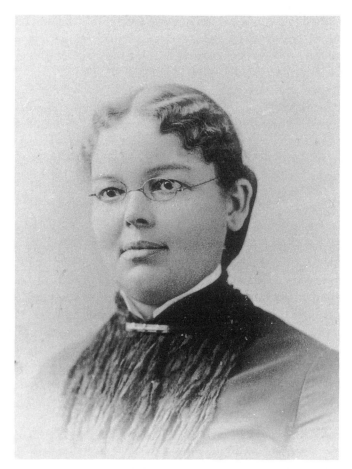

Figure 2. Ida V. Smith. (By permission of Mount Holyoke College; courtesy of Mount Holyoke College Archives)

this expectation imposes current standards on the nineteenth century. Discourse then was more circumspect, and Richards, a woman of her times, seemed to expect the WBM to read between her lines: "The home friends do not realize how little one can do till we get so we can use our tongues. It is trying to the new ones particularly. They want so much to do all they see being done. . . . [I]t is surely very trying [to] work through an interpretor [*sic*]. They do not half understand and so they make all sorts of mistakes in interpreting and do not hear the strangest things that we have told the people. . . . If we could only realize this when we first come and not rush

too fast into things we cannot do. But take things easily and wait till we can speak, we would have many less mistakes and be of very much more use to the people." There was need for more missionaries but, said Richards, "old missionaries are the ones doing the work which tells."[81]

Meanwhile, Smith put a very different spin on the same experience. She told the WBM that Richards was in excellent health and trusted that she "may be enabled to assist her so that she will not be sick again. We are very happy altogether. She is much more self-reliant than I ever expect to be. I find I am a child in many ways."[82] Later that year a more openly angry Smith disparaged Richards's responsibilities, saying that Richards was apparently not "over-burdened with work."[83]

Womanly Wisdom Wasted

Richards was a good judge of character, according to those who had recommended her for missionary work. Surely her close work with women as superintendent of training schools in Boston had honed this skill. She and Denton caught onto Smith's duplicity long before Berry did. Some of Smith's cleverness is evident in the sharply contrasting pictures Richards and Berry drew. Richards told Berry that she could not put the work into Smith's incompetent and careless hands. Berry, by contrast, praised Smith, who he thought would develop into a fine worker. The power of Smith's strategy is also evidenced in Berry's being troubled by Richards's behavior toward Smith, stating that Richards was peremptory and unjust. Richards criticized and condemned Smith, said Berry, rather than bear with little things and counsel her to overcome them as a senior associate should.[84]

Berry was an unwitting ploy in the struggle, though in fairness to the man, perhaps Smith showed him only her good side. Women, however, were on to Smith. For example, a visitor to the mission immediately picked up Smith's style saying, "You cannot stab a person one minute and caress her the next."[85] Another overheard Smith saying that the ABCFM had sent her out to take Richards's position. Indeed, said Smith, she had not come to Japan to be second to anyone.[86] This was completely counter to the ABCFM's direction. They had advised Smith that she would naturally defer to Miss Richards as the head of the institution and underscored how she was prepared for this position with "special training and experience."[87] This advice, as all the advice to come, rolled off Smith. Although the women had more than enough data on the negative aspects of Smith's behavior and were also in the majority, Berry's input carried the more weight. Consequently, Smith continued on a course leading to the destruction not only of

the training school, but also the relationship between the DoShisha and the ABCFM.

Alienated from Richards and the single women missionaries, Smith turned to the students in the training school. She apparently encouraged the opposition to the school which had never abated, though it had become quiescent. Aided and abetted by the vengeful missionary wife, Smith stirred up suspicious Japanese. Then she told the students that Richards was an ignorant woman who not only knew nothing of nursing but was working the students too hard. Students in the United States only oversaw the work of others, said Smith. Furthermore, she continued, Richards was demanding the students do work that she herself could not do.

Four nurses left the hospital for the school at Tokyo but not before they criticized Richards's methods and manners. She could not understand how nurses who had once been so kind to her could now be so hostile. Making difficulties worse, some of these students had been educated at the expense of donations raised by Richards's friends in Somerville, Massachusetts. Richards felt first humiliated by and then terrified of the angry students, a shame and a fear that were exacerbated by her own disappointment and exhaustion.[88]

At this point, Richards wanted to resign her position and give the school to Smith. Richards's associates urged her not to quit, especially Denton, perhaps self-interestedly, because she did not want to work with Smith. Berry was entirely unprepared for the tumult. He seemed to take the information at face value and did not explore its deeper meaning. At the mission meeting held to discuss the problems, he broke the tied vote — three missionaries for Richards and three for Smith — in favor of Richards. "As Miss Richards had borne the labor of the first years of work and was the senior, it was but just that she have the choice in the matter," wrote Berry in August 1889, damning Richards with faint praise.[89] Berry had had some minor differences with Richards over the training school, but he always supported her work and defended her to the ABCFM. He must have known that Richards had worked well with other women in the mission and was esteemed by all of them except for Smith and the disgruntled missionary wife. It is hard to explain why Berry was not more vigorous in his support of Richards.

Given only two options by Boston, Smith chose to go to Niigata to teach in the Boys' School rather than go home, which would have been a public acknowledgment of failure.[90] Even as she left for Niigata, however, Smith declared that she wanted to return to the training school for which

she had prepared herself "by many years of careful study and which [she] came to Japan expressly to practice."[91] Berry remained in the dark about Smith, especially her furious vows to ruin Richards. He continued to feel "very sorry for Miss Smith."[92] When she left for Niigata in October, too quickly as events would show, the ABCFM decided that the trouble had been adjusted and was no longer a source of anxiety.

Once in Niigata, Smith kept up her attack on Richards. Smith drew a picture of Richards rejecting her as a companion and associate and ignoring her socially and professionally. In words echoing Berry's sentiments about Richards, Smith continued: "Miss Richards, as my senior associate, instead of going to the other members of the station and even writing to you seeking to injure my reputation, [should have] come to me in a spirit of Christian love and told me wherein I had been at fault. But this she has never done."[93]

Richards continued in Kyoto for only a short time longer. She no longer had the will to fight, especially now because she feared the Japanese. She resigned her position as head of the training school on 27 February 1890, but before it could take effect, in June 1890, she came down with a cold and required prolonged rest in Shanghai. The doctors in the hospital succeeded Richards and helped the students complete their term. Throughout all the tumult—the mission vote, Berry's unswerving confidence in Smith, the departure of Smith for Niigata, and Richards's resignation—the ABCFM retained its trust in Richards. Clarke told Berry, "I have always felt very just confidence in [Richards] — in her spirit — charity and self-denying devotion to every good work." At the same time, he was a "good deal exercised by the case of Miss Smith" and was wary of the "doubts and difficulties affecting her character of a serious nature." He hoped, however, that Richards would continue in Japan, if not with the training school.[94]

The resignation brought Smith, Richards's only possible successor, once again to Kyoto. Tales of her alienating her missionary colleagues in Niigata and going deeply in debt preceded her return. Clark wrote that it would be better to close the school than to allow Smith to be a burden and annoyance to the mission.[95] This option was discounted because, by this time, the missionaries considered it a practical and tangible charity that was "one of the most important avenues to [their] work in Japan."[96] They knew that patients who had been helped at the hospital were favorably predisposed to hear the Gospel from a worker who had cared for them.

Just as it looked as though the tumult over the training school had quieted, Nee-Sima died. With the death of "the father of Japanese educa-

tion," Boston's hopes of a great spiritual awakening were quickly squelched as natives gave unrestrained voice to the fury Nee-Sima once held in check. The tenuous relationship between the Japanese and the mission was maintained, although Richards believed Berry accomplished this by disparaging her as an old, outdated teacher and praising Smith's youth and new ideas. How much of this was true, and not just Richards's disappointment, is hard to say at this remove. But there is no doubt that Berry was firmly, if blindly, still on Smith's side. "Personally," he wrote, "I have never seen anything in Miss Smith's character or manner to disqualify her for the position." He was surprised but open to the reports from Niigata that were "decidedly derogatory to [Smith]."[97] He would be enlightened still more as he tried to manage Smith during the next year. None of this touched Smith who happily reported, "I am back in Kyoto in the work I came to Japan [to do]."[98]

Eliza Talcott (1836–1911), the wise woman of the mission, was pressed into service ostensibly to be an associate, but her real job was to keep a tight rein on Smith. Talcott praised Smith's enthusiasm for her work but worried that she had not gained enough control of herself that the position required. "I am sure," said Talcott, "she does not realize the extent of the evil her example is having on those around her, an evil all the more insidious because she has such recognized talent." Talcott stopped there, feeling she would be disloyal to Smith if she discussed "her peculiarities."[99] As the year progressed, however, "impatient," "impetuous," "insufficient self-discipline," "ambitious," "jealous," and "untruthful" were some of the terms used to describe Smith. Meanwhile, the woman who was driving many people to distraction reported that she was as "happy as the day was long." In fact, she had never been so well in her life. She had a good appetite, slept well, and weighed 176 pounds of "good solid flesh."[100]

Clarke, Berry, and Talcott got Smith through the year, though often with great difficulty. Still, Smith was not without her talents. She was a good teacher, but her character, the aspect of nursing that the mission was trying to mold in their Japanese students, was incorrigible. Talcott said Smith "did not mean to misrepresent. She has a strong imagination and somehow her statements need verification."[101] By March, Berry wanted Smith to go home, though he could not say that to her directly without incurring another upheaval. Essentially, neither he nor Talcott trusted Smith, and all through that year Berry and Clarke looked for a successor. When the year was over, Berry advised Smith to resign. She was completely taken by surprise, but recovered enough to retaliate. She accused Talcott, whom she

had once described as "gold, pure gold," of duplicity and failure to inform her of faults that might have been corrected. Unlike the earlier triangle, when Smith relied on Berry in her attack on Richards, an enlightened Berry stood staunchly with Talcott and not Smith. Furthermore, this time Smith had no allies in the mission. When she tried to persuade Clarke of the righteousness of her cause, she found she was alone there, too. "I am sorry to say that I have other testimony less favorable to you," wrote Clarke, "and of such a character as makes me feel anxious in reference to your happy continuance in the field."[102] The mission learned by harsh experience what they might have gained had it listened to Richards and other single women missionaries. Its vote to accept Smith's resignation was unanimous.[103]

Richards Quenches Her Little Torch

During the year that Richards was in Shanghai trying to recover from physical exhaustion and mental strain, Clarke wrote to her often, reassuring her that she had not made a mistake in going to Japan and focusing her instead on the fact that she had won the respect and esteem and hearty Christian regard of all.[104] Such support could not relieve Richards of the memory of the Japanese nurses turning on her or her disappointment in the nurses. "They do almost no Christian work," complained Richards, "They work for money." Furthermore, Richards was crushed that she was succeeded by a woman like Smith who could still injure Richards's good name in Japan. "Forty such women as she could not harm me among those I know at home," wrote Richards, nor could Smith ever have gained a "position of trust in the United States."[105] Clarke had already advised Richards not to dwell on this and directed her to consider her accomplishments:

> Who could have taken up the work which you have done in Kyoto? Who could have made such a success of the Nurses School? Who [could] have won such esteem and regard for it? Who could have laid foundations for the training of thousands of nurses in years to come? Who could have contributed to the welfare and happiness of tens of thousands of Japanese during the coming decades? . . . We have only one Miss Richards in all Japan. Yours is a missionary work in planting an institution which in its wide influence is to reach in the coming years to a vastly greater number than you could possibly hope to reach at home. It is not a question of ministering to the wants of ten, or a hundred persons. It is not a matter of just now, but of prospective influence in years to come. I beg . . . that you will not allow yourself to be troubled by any unfavorable comments that may be made touching your work . . . but quietly and cheerfully accept the opportunity of wide influence which is opening to you.[106]

RICHARDS FACES WEST

But Richards knew her time in Japan was over, and with each letter to Boston she asked to be released from her commitment. Even as Richards left Japan, Clarke wrote of her: "We have a high appreciation of her work in Japan. She did faithful work in connection with the School and Hospital for Nurses according to the best of her ability. She was ready at any time to enter upon special duties. . . . She has shown a self-sacrificing spirit very much to our admiration."[107]

During this same time, too, the DoShisha grew more and more hostile to the mission. The Reverend Mr. H. Kozaki, Nee-Sima's successor, stated that the time had come for the trustees to decide whether the hospital belonged to Berry or the DoShisha. Berry argued that he took charge because the trustees had utterly neglected their duties to the hospital, but this did not influence the trustees of the DoShisha.[108] The civil authorities had protested at the beginning because the training school was headed by a foreigner. Now with both Richards and Nee-Sima gone, the Japanese took control of the school.

If the training school and its hospital were in jeopardy, so too was the relationship between the ABCFM and the DoShisha. The ABCFM had contributed thousands of dollars to establish the DoShisha in 1875 and had generously supported it in the intervening fifteen years. Increasingly, the DoShisha was adding sciences and math to the curriculum, making it more a secular institution and less a Christian missionary school. Such a secular drift had carried Harvard, the DoShisha's exemplar, from its moorings, worried Clark in Boston.[109] He was sensitive to these changes and worried about the rumbling discord between the DoShisha and the missionaries. He advised them to have their passports near at hand in case they would need to show they were American citizens and entitled to protection. He advised missionaries everywhere to be very careful and to obey the rules and regulations of the government.[110]

The relationship of the DoShisha with the mission continued to deteriorate, though there was an uneasy truce for the next five years. Helen Fraser (1868–?), of Toronto, Canada, a graduate of the Bellevue Hospital School of Nursing, worked with Miss Talcott during this time though the "lack of cordiality among the Japanese [made] work extremely difficult."[111] Much as Richards was given kudos from the Japanese for her offer to care for cholera victims, Fraser, Berry, and the school were praised for their heroic efforts during the 28 October 1891 earthquake in Gifu. Sympathy peaked for the training school, but these positive feelings lasted only a short time. On 10 June 1896, the school closed after the last class completed its

courses. Berry left Japan on vacation in 1893 expecting to return; however, Japanese nationalism fully exerted itself at the DoShisha and he was no longer welcome.

Conclusion

Richards's dream of converting heathen women turned into a nightmare, but her school did succeed in graduating its first four trained nurses on 26 June 1888. Seventy-five nurses eventually graduated from the training school in Kyoto before it closed in 1896. Richards's successor remarked, "[The graduates] are scattered all over the country, most of them doing excellent work and whatever the future of the school may be, their work must go on and their influence be far-reaching. That cannot be hindered or stopped."[112] As Clarke had prophesied, Richards's first four graduates in the class of 1888 became a "prospective influence in years to come." One hundred years after Richards left Japan, there are 652,000 nurses in Japan.[113]

A NEW MISSION FOR RICHARDS
Two years after Richards returned to the United States, the Congress of Missions reported on its century-long exportation of Protestant Christianity. Nurses were at the Chicago World's Fair of 1893, too, and presented at the International Congress of Charities, Corrections and Philanthropy. Among the papers was one from Richards on her experience in missionary nursing. She was silent about the childhood dreams, the adolescent spirituality, and the adult religious reawakening that had taken her to the Far East. Nor did she speak of the tumult and heartache of her work with other single women missionaries and the cost of the Protestant feminism they pioneered.[114] That same week, nurses created the American Society of Superintendents of Training Schools for Nurses (precursor of the National League for Nursing Education and the National League for Nursing). Richards became its first president, and as the millennium edged closer, she began a new mission. For the next forty years, often fretting about her health, Richards cemented her role as "America's first trained nurse," the tangible symbol of the nursing profession.

MARY ELLEN DOONA, EdD, RN
Associate Professor
Boston College
Chestnut Hill, MA 02167
Phone: (617) 552-4269

Acknowledgments

This article was supported by a Boston College Research Expense Grant.

Notes

1. George Tuttle to ABCFM, 24 August 1885. In Linda Richards, Candidates R-V, American Board of Commissioners of Foreign Missions — Japan Mission, Harvard College Houghton Library (hereafter cited as ABCFM-JM). Used by permission of the Houghton Library and United Church Board for World Ministries (successor to ABCFM).

2. George Beard, "Neurasthenia or Nervous Exhaustion," *Boston Medical and Surgical Journal* (1869): 217–21.

3. Jean Strouse, *Alice James: A Biography* (Boston: Houghton Mifflin Co., 1980), xiv.

4. The enforced rest treatment was created by neurologist/novelist, S. Weir Mitchell. See the critique of the treatment in Charlotte Perkins Gilman, *The Yellow Wallpaper* (New York: Feminist Press, 1973).

5. Linda Richards, 21 August 1885, Candidates R-V, ABCFM-JM.

6. Richards, Candidates R-V, ABCFM-JM.

7. Barbara Welter, "She Hath Done What She Could: Protestant Women's Missionary Careers in Nineteenth-Century America," in *Women in American Religious History,* ed. Janet Wilson James (Philadelphia: University of Pennsylvania Press, 1980), 111–25; and Mrs. Potter Palmer, "President of the Woman's Branch of the World Congress Auxiliary of the Women's Department of the World Columbian Exposition," in *Christian Practicality* (New York: Baker and Taylor, 1894), 10–11.

8. Richards, Candidates R-V, ABCFM-JM.

9. Stella Goostray, "Linda Richards," in *Notable American Women,* ed. Edward James and Janet W. James (Cambridge, Mass.: Belknap Press of Harvard University Press, 1972), 148–50.

10. John C. Berry to N. G. Clarke, 14 May 1885, Letters from Missionaries (hereafter cited as LM), ABCFM-JM.

11. N. G. Clarke to John C. Berry, 3 December 1885, Letters to Foreign Missions, ABCFM-JM.

12. Richards, Candidates R-V, ABCFM-JM.

13. Helen Barrett Montgomery, *Western Women in Eastern Lands* (New York: Macmillan, 1910; reprint, New York: Garland Publishing, 1987), 243.

14. Minutes of the Women's Board of Missions, 2 January 1868 and 3 November 1868, ABCFM-JM (hereafter cited as WBM).

15. WBM, 2 January 1868.

16. WBM, 15 June 1885.

17. WBM, 15 November 1885; John J. McCusker, "How Much Is That in Real Money: A Historical Price Index for Use as a Deflator of Money Values in the Economy of the United States," *Proceedings of the American Antiquarian Society* 101 (part II, 1992): 297–373.

18. Mrs. Frank Tyler to E. K. Alden, n.d., Candidates R-V, ABCFM-JM.

19. Mary Prescott to E. K. Alden, 24 August 1855, Candidates R-V, ABCFM-JM.

20. Edward Cowles to E. K. Alden, 24 August 1885, Candidates R-V, ABCFM-JM.

21. George Rowe to E. K. Alden, 25 August 1885, Candidates R-V, ABCFM-JM.

22. Morris J. Vogel, *The Invention of the Modern Hospital: Boston 1870–1930* (Chicago: University of Chicago, 1980), 40.

23. John C. Berry to N. G. Clarke, 12 August 1885, Candidates R-V, ABCFM-JM.

24. In 1875 Richards earned $900 annually at the Boston Training School. Minutes of the Board of Directors, Boston Training School, September 1874, Collection of the Massachusetts General Hospital School of Nursing, Harvard College Francis A. Countway Library, Boston, p. 89.

25. Linda Richards to E. K. Alden, 8 September 1885, Candidates R-V, ABCFM-JM.

26. Another view of this era is offered in Ellen D. Baer, "Nursing's Divided House — An Historical View," *Nursing Research* (January/February, 1985): 32–38.

27. Linda Richards to WBM, 27 January 1886, LM, ABCFM-JM.

28. Linda Richards to My dear Emeline [Masta Davis], 21 August 1886, The New England Hospital for Women and Children Collection, Smithsonian Institution (hereafter cited as NEHWC). Richards lived as a child with the Masta family in Vermont. This family, of Somerville, Massachusetts, during Richards's Japan experience raised money to support Japanese nursing students.

29. Linda Richards to WBM, 27 January 1886, LM, ABCFM-JM.

30. Linda Richards to N. G. Clarke, 28 January 1886, LM, ABCFM-JM.

31. John Berry to N. G. Clarke, 20 April 1886, ABCFM-JM.

32. N. G. Clarke to Linda Richards, 8 September 1886, LM, ABCFM.

33. Linda Richards to Emeline [Masta Davis], 21 August 1886, NEHWC.

34. John C. Berry to N. G. Clarke, 26 August 1886, LM, ABCFM-JM. See also John C. Berry Journal, 118–31, ABCFM-JM; and John C. Berry, "A Christian Training School for Nurses in Kioto," *Light and Life* 15 (1885): 375–77.

35. Frank A. Lombard, *A History of the Japan Mission of the American Board* (ABCFM): 3, 13.

36. *Hiogo News,* 26 May 1886, cited in Lombard, *The DoShisha,* ABCFM-JM.

37. Joseph H. Nee-Sima, 11 June 1886, in John C. Berry Journal, 129–30, ABCFM-JM.

38. Linda Richards to N. G. Clark, 20 October 1886, LM, ABCFM-JM.

39. Linda Richards to N. G. Clarke, 21 September 1886, LM, ABCFM-JM.

40. Linda Richards to WMB, 14 March 1887, LM, ABCFM-JM.

41. Linda Richards to N. G. Clarke, 21 September 1886, LM, ABCFM-JM.

42. Linda Richards to WBM, 14 March 1887, and to N. G. Clarke, 2 February 1887 and 17 February 1887, LM, ABCFM-JM.

43. Linda Richards to WBM, 25 October 1888, LM, ABCFM-JM.

44. Linda Richards to WBM, 7 May 1888, LM, ABCFM-JM.

45. John C. Berry to N. G. Clarke, 27 September 1886 and 28 December 1886, LM, ABCFM-JM.

46. Abbie B. Child to Linda Richards, 9 June 1887, ABCFM-JM.

47. Linda Richards to My dear Ida, 18 March 1888, LM, NEHWC, and to WBM, 14 March 1887, LM, ABCFM-JM.

48. Linda Richards to WBM, 17 February 1887, LM, ABCFM-JM.

49. N. G. Clarke to Linda Richards, 10 June 1887, LM, ABCFM-JM.

50. Sara Craig Buckley to N. G. Clarke, 27 May 1887, LM, ABCFM-JM.

51. Linda Richards to WBM, 22 June 1887, LM, ABCFM-JM.

52. Linda Richards to WBM, 25 October 1888, LM, ABCFM-JM.

53. Ibid.

54. WBM, 5 July 1887, ABCFM-JM.

55. Linda Richards to WBM, 5 November 1887, LM, ABCFM-JM.

56. Linda Richards to WBM, 24 July 1888, LM, ABCFM-JM.

57. Linda Richards to My dear Emeline [Masta Davis], 1 January 1889, NEHWC.

58. Linda Richards to WBM, 25 October 1888, LM, ABCFM-JM.

59. John C. Berry to N. G. Clarke, 25 May 1888, LM, ABCFM-JM.

60. Linda Richards to N. G. Clarke, 23 December 1887, LM, NEHWC.

61. Sara Craig Buckley to WBM, n.d. March 1887 and 22 October 1887, LM, ABCFM-JM.

62. Sara Craig Buckley to WBM, 11 November 1887 and 24 January 1888, LM, ABCFM-JM.

63. John C. Berry to N. G. Clarke, 30 March 1888, LM, ABCFM-JM.

64. Linda Richards to WBM, 23 January 1888, and to N. G. Clarke, 23 January 1888, LM, ABCFM-JM.

65. Flora Denton to WBM, 31 July 1888, LM, ABCFM-JM.

66. Flora Denton to WBM, 14 November 1888, LM, ABCFM-JM.

67. Janet Wilson James, "Women in American Religious History: An Overview," in *Women in American Religious History* (Philadelphia: University of Pennsylvania Press, 1980).

68. Flora Denton to WBM, 12 June 1889, LM, ABCFM-JM.

69. Linda Richards to WBM, 24 July 1888, and to N. G. Clarke, 25 October 1888, LM, ABCFM-JM.

70. Linda Richards, 25 October 1888, LM, WBM.

71. Sara Craig Buckley to N. G. Clark, 5 September 1888, LM, ABCFM-JM.

72. Linda Richards to N. G. Clarke, 14 February 1888, 16 April 1888, 24 May 1888, and to WBM, 25 October 1888, LM, ABCFM-JM.

73. Linda Richards to WBM, 7 May 1888, and to N. G. Clarke, 23 January 1888, LM, ABCFM-JM.

74. N. G. Clarke to Linda Richards, 3 December 1888, ABCFM-JM.

75. Linda Richards to WBM, 3 December 1888, and to N. G. Clarke, 4 January 1889, LM, ABCFM-JM.

76. Linda Richards to WBM, 19 November 1888, LM, ABCFM-JM.

77. John C. Berry to N. G. Clarke, 11 February 1889, LM, ABCFM-JM.

78. John C. Berry to N. G. Clarke, 24 February 1889, LM, ABCFM-JM.

79. Ida V. Smith to Miss Hill, WBM, 1 February 1888, LM, ABCFM-JM.

80. Ida V. Smith to Miss Hill, WBM, 13 March 1888, LM, ABCFM-JM.

81. Linda Richards to WBM, 16 March 1889, LM, ABCFM-JM.

82. Ida V. Smith to N. G. Clarke, 13 March 1889, LM, ABCFM-JM.

83. Ida V. Smith to N. G. Clarke, 30 August 1889, LM, ABCFM-JM.

84. John C. Berry to N. G. Clarke, 15 August 1889, LM, ABCFM-JM.

85. Eliza Talcott to WBM to N. G. Clarke, 23 July 1889, LM, ABCFM-JM.

86. Linda Richards to N. G. Clarke, 19 July 1890, LM, ABCFM-JM.

87. N. G. Clarke to Ida V. Smith, 15 May 1889, ABCFM-JM.

88. Linda Richards to N. G. Clarke, 19 July 1890; John C. Berry to N. G. Clarke, 25 March 1890, LM, ABCFM-JM.

89. John C. Berry to N. G. Clarke, 15 August 1889, LM, ABCFM-JM.

90. N. G. Clarke to Ida V. Smith, 22 July 1889, ABCFM-JM.

91. Ida V. Smith to N. G. Clarke, 30 August 1889, LM, ABCFM-JM.

92. John C. Berry to N. G. Clarke, 15 August 1889, LM, ABCFM-JM.

93. Ida V. Smith, 30 August 1889.

94. N. G. Clarke to John C. Berry, 9 April 1890, 26 April 1890, ABCFM-JM.

95. N. G. Clarke to Arthur Stanford, 28 March 1890, ABCFM-JM.

96. Arthur Stanford to N. G. Clarke, 19 May 1890, LM, ABCFM-JM.

97. John C. Berry to N. G. Clarke, 19 April 1890, LM, ABCFM-JM.

98. Ida V. Smith to Mrs. Clarke, 17 November 1890, LM, ABCFM-JM.

99. Eliza Talcott to N. G. Clarke, 5 June 1889, LM, ABCFM-JM.

100. Ida V. Smith to [WBM], 18 April 1891, LM, ABCFM-JM.

101. Eliza Talcott to Miss Child, 23 July 1891, LM, ABCFM-JM.

102. N. G. Clarke to Ida V. Smith, 13 May 1891, LM, ABCFM-JM.

103. John C. Berry to N. G. Clarke, 30 July 1891, LM, ABCFM-JM.

104. N. G. Clarke to Linda Richards, 19 February 1890, ABCFM-JM.

105. Linda Richards to N. G. Clarke, 19 July 1890, LM, ABCFM-JM.

106. N. G. Clarke to Linda Richards, 19 February 1890, ABCFM-JM.

107. N. G. Clarke to Arthur Stanford, 21 August 1890, LM, ABCFM-JM.

108. John C. Berry to N. G. Clarke, 29 May 1890, LM, ABCFM-JM.

109. N. G. Clarke to Arthur Stanford, 31 October 1890, ABCFM-JM.

110. N. G. Clarke to D. W. Learned, 9 December 1890, and to Arthur Stanford, 11 June 1890, ABCFM-JM.

111. Helen Fraser to WBM, 12 December 1891, LM, ABCFM-JM.

112. Helen Fraser to N. G. Clarke, 15 April 1896, ABCFM-JM.

113. *World Health Statistics Annual* (Geneva: World Health Organization 1988).

114. Linda Richards, "Mission Training Schools and Nursing," in *Hospitals, Dispensaries and Nursing*, ed. John S. Billings and Henry M. Hurd (Baltimore: Johns Hopkins University Press, 1894), 565–69.

Missionaries and the Early Development of Nursing in China

Kaiyi Chen
University Archives
University of Pennsylvania

Nursing, along with modern Western medicine, was introduced to China by Western medical missionaries. In the absence of trained nurses in the earliest days, medical missionary pioneers tried to provide makeshift nursing service with unskilled temporary Chinese assistants at their clinics and dispensaries. Elizabeth McKechnie, a graduate nurse from the Woman's Hospital of Philadelphia, was the first Western-trained nurse to come to China.[1] On her arrival in Shanghai in 1884, Miss McKechnie joined Dr. Elizabeth Reifsnyder, a surgeon of the American Women's Union Missionary Society and a graduate from the Woman's Medical College of Pennsylvania. They ran a small dispensary in Shanghai near a place called West Gate.[2] According to the existing records, the Woman's Hospital of Philadelphia established the first chartered nurses training school of North America in 1863. It was only some twenty years later that the seed of modern nursing was transplanted from America to China.[3]

The last two decades of the nineteenth century saw a surge of missionary enthusiasm in both North America and England. By 1887, as many as seventy-four Western medical missionaries, thirty-three British and forty-one Americans were working in different parts of China.[4] As knowledge of modern Western medicine grew, China experienced an increasing demand for medical personnel. Under these circumstances, the training of Chinese doctors and nurses became highly desirable. In presenting the first issue of the *China Medical Missionary Journal,* Dr. John G. Kerr, president of the Medical Missionary Association of China, claimed that medical education had become "a legitimate department" of missionary work. Missionaries, he asserted, "will do no less good" in training native physicians and nurses than in ministering directly to the sick in hospitals, dispensaries, or at the

Nursing History Review 4 (1996): 129–49. Copyright © 1996 by The American Association for the History of Nursing.

bedside.[5] In the same issue, Dr. Henry W. Boone, an American Protestant Episcopal Church Mission doctor who had been in charge of St. Luke's Hospital in Shanghai since 1880, also vehemently appealed to his colleagues to "set ourselves to train up a body of skilled nurses."[6]

Formative Years of Nursing Schools: 1887–1914

The training of Chinese nurses began in a few missionary hospitals in coastal cities of China. In 1887, Dr. Boone reported that at St. Luke's Hospital, "one man and one woman are under special instruction to fit them for the performances of the duties of trained nurses."[7] In Nanking, another coastal city in central China, Miss Esther H. Butler, a missionary of the American Friends Mission and a graduate of the Chicago Training School, started nurses' training in 1888.[8] In the same year, Miss Ella Johnson started a training class of nursing girls in Foochow, a coastal city in south China. Toward the end of the century, Dr. Lillie E. V. Saville of the London Missionary Society started a class for nursing and dispensing in Peking.[9] In 1896, a school named after an American benefactor, Mrs. Julia M. Turner, developed a two-year nursing program in Canton. Following guidelines provided by Isabel Adams Hampton in *Nursing: Its Principles and Practice,* pupils at the Canton school were taught courses such as ethics of nursing; hygiene; materia medica; anatomy and physiology; general lectures on medicine, surgery, obstetrics, and gynecology; contagious and infectious diseases; care of children; and massage.[10] In 1889, Dr. Boone reported as president of the Medical Missionary Association that throughout the empire, from Manchuria in the northeast to Canton in the south, while male medical missionaries were busy teaching and training male medical pupils, women doctors had begun the good work of training women doctors and nurses.[11]

Given the great disparity between modern Western culture and old Chinese traditions at that time, it is not difficult to imagine the hardship and frustrations early missionary doctors and nurses experienced in China. To adapt themselves to local conditions, missionaries had to work hard to learn the Chinese language and, in some cases, the local dialect, too. Gradually, they would also pick up some Chinese ways of living appropriate to their status in the local community.[12] But despite the increasing acceptance by the Chinese society of the value of Western medicine, the deeply seated mistrust of the natives, combined with the varying degrees of superiority

betrayed inadvertently or otherwise by missionaries themselves as both authorities on Christian gospels and representatives of Western civilization, prevented the missionaries from fully mixing with the Chinese. Missionaries and their families, therefore, kept living in isolation within their own compounds, a hardship that the relative affluence and influence they generally enjoyed could hardly compensate for.[13]

Missions in some interior provinces fared even worse. From 1888 to 1899, for instance, the Presbyterian Church in Canada sent to Honan Province, central China, twenty-four missionaries, among them eight physicians and four registered nurses. Since seven missionaries came with their spouses and some with children as well, the number of the entire missionary community totaled forty. In quite a few localities, the Canadian missionaries encountered suspicion and hostility from the local people. In 1891, the mission actually had one of its working stations looted. Partly because of inadequate living and medical conditions, three missionaries and ten children died in the thirteen years the mission operated in the province. When the Boxer Rebellion took shape in the early summer of 1900, all the personnel were evacuated after a warning from the British Consul in Tientsin, and the Canadian Church formally closed the mission in July of that year.[14]

By the turn of the century, the government of the Ching Court, having lost its war with the Allied Powers in the Boxer Movement upheaval, was compelled to be more tolerant of Western ideas and influences. In the meantime, the new open-door policy for China advocated by the U.S. government further encouraged the interest of Western missionaries. Under such circumstances, the training of nurses gathered momentum. Efforts to start or consolidate nursing programs were reported in many coastal cities. In Peking, the London Mission joined forces with the American Presbyterian and Methodist Missions and opened the Union School for Nurses in October 1906. Dr. Saville abolished the prevalent practice of allowing mothers and friends to live with the patients in the hospital and provided uniforms for the nurses. When the London Missionary Society withdrew in 1908, the two American missions carried on.[15] In Tientsin, Dr. Yamei Kin, the first Chinese woman physician trained abroad, opened a school for nurses with the aid of a grant from the viceroy of the province Yuan Shi-k'ai.[16] In Nanking, a Union Nurses' Home and School opened its doors at the Friends' Hospital in October 1908.[17] A little later, nurses' training started at hospitals sponsored by the American Presbyterian Mission in two smaller coastal cities — Chefoo, Shantung Province, and Soochow, a city not far from Shanghai. The Temple Hill Hospital at Chefoo

reported in 1917 that of its first three nursing graduates, two remained at the hospital, one in charge of the operating room and one to act as technician in the laboratory, while the third started to work at a hospital in the biggest seaport of the province. The quality of the students was reported to be satisfactory.[18] The requirement for admission at one Presbyterian hospital in Soochow was remarkably liberal. Anyone who had learned "enough Chinese to use the text book" would be eligible.[19] Farther south, the Magaw Memorial Hospital in Foochow reorganized its training of nurses and established the Florence Nightingale Nurses' Training School in 1909.

In Canton, the Julia M. Turner Training School for Nurses became affiliated in 1902 with two Presbyterian missionary institutions: the David Gregg Hospital for Women and the Hackett Medical College for Women. Presumably because of the limited pool of women applicants, the school set its entrance requirement at two years of study in Chinese and Chinese writing.[20] For a text, Dr. Mary H. Fulton, founder of the Turner School and the two other Presbyterian institutions, translated into Chinese *Nursing in Abdominal Surgery and Diseases of Women,* a work by Anna M. Fullerton, MD, of Philadelphia.[21]

Also in Canton, the University Medical School sponsored by the Christian Association of the University of Pennsylvania started a nursing school in October 1911. Dr. William W. Cadbury, a missionary doctor partially supported by the Christian Association, undertook the training of three male nurses and two female nurses. The training comprised practical experience in medical and surgical nursing as well as lectures on anatomy, physiology, and practical nursing. After a period of training, the nursing students were admitted to the staff on two months' probation.[22] By 1914, the training had grown into a three-year program for an enrollment of ten Chinese nursing students, five women and five men. The school, managed by an American matron, Mrs. M. S. Macher (a graduate nurse of the Bryn Mawr Hospital near Philadelphia), was believed to be then the only school in all China where male nurses were as "fully trained" as female nurses.[23]

This period saw nursing education spread to various parts of inland China as well. In Hankow, central China, an English nurse helped begin the training of male nurses in the city's Men's Hospital.[24] In the neighboring city of Wuchang, the Wesleyan mission opened a nurses' training school around the turn of the century. Under the Wesleyan mission's influence, Dr. Mary Glanton, together with a nurse, Miss Susan B. Higgins, a graduate of the Philadelphia General Hospital Nurse Training School, started in 1907 another nurses' training program at the Elizabeth Bunn Memorial Hospital

in the same city.[25] Nurses' training developed even in the remote south-western part of China. In Chungking, for instance, the General Hospital of the Methodist Episcopal Mission in 1902 admitted three young men for a three-year course in nursing instruction.[26]

The best known and most formally organized medical missionary effort, however, was to be found in Changsha, Hunan province.[27] A student missionary society at Yale University had begun sending missionaries to the city in central China at the turn of the century. In 1906, the mission established a hospital. Three years later, Nina D. Gage, a 1905 graduate of the Wellesley College and registered nurse of the Roosevelt Hospital of New York City, joined the Yale mission at Changsha. After spending her first year exclusively studying Chinese, Miss Gage established a nurses' training program as part of the Yale mission there in 1910. She gave five Chinese nurses, four male and one female, both theoretical and practical instruction. The training soon developed into two separate nursing schools, one for men and one for women.[28] Miss Gage was so successful in systematizing the training program at the Yale-in-China hospital that during her absence in the winter of 1911–1912, the Chinese nurses were able to carry on the work of the elaborate system by themselves. When the two nursing schools formally opened in December 1913, they had a total enrollment of fifty-four students, of which forty were men and fourteen women.[29]

To meet the needs of an increasing number of newly trained Chinese nurses, a little handbook — *Manual of Nursing* — was published by the Medical Missionary Association of China in 1906. The manual covered general science subjects, such as anatomy and physiology, as well as nursing procedures for all areas — medical, surgical, obstetric, and pediatric. It also had a glossary of terms in English and Chinese.[30]

The Birth of the Nurses' Association of China

As nursing education burgeoned across the land in the first decade of the century, some leading missionary nurses in China met at Kuling, a summer mountain resort in Kiangsi Province, in the summers of 1908 and 1909. The participants, representing areas where nursing had first developed in China, organized themselves as the Nurses' Association of China (NAC). The purpose of the NAC was, in addition to promoting fellowship among its members for mutual help, to raise the standard of nurses' training in China by the adoption of "a uniform course of study and examination."[31] The new

organization, though having then only a membership of ten foreign nurses plus one or two Chinese nurses, signaled the coming of a new and increasingly mature stage of the nursing profession in China.[32]

For the first couple of years, the NAC was loosely organized and somewhat uncertain in its direction. Shortly after the 1911 revolution turned the ancient empire into a republic, missionary nursing leaders met again in Kuling in 1912 and 1913, encouraged by a nationwide revived interest in reforms and learning from the West. The NAC was reorganized, and Miss Gage was elected president, a position she was to hold until 1914. The participants at those meetings resolved that in the absence of uniform government authority on nursing education, the NAC should take into its own hands such matters as setting a standard for all nursing schools in the country, formulating a model curriculum, and holding certification examinations.[33] At the 1912 meeting, it was decided to convene a national convention in Shanghai in 1914.

The Shanghai conference gave the honor of chairmanship to Miss Elsie Mawfung Chung, a 1909 graduate from Guy's Hospital, London, and the first Chinese nurse ever trained abroad. As there had been no equivalent for the word "nurse" in Chinese, Miss Chung, after consulting a number of Sinologues, chose one out of several Chinese versions. The Chinese term *hu-shih* is made up of two Chinese characters:

$$護 \quad 士$$

The first one, *hu,* carries the meaning of "protection" or "care," while the second one, *shih,* means "scholar" or "technician." The Chinese translation of the name of the NAC was simultaneously set. Exercising its authority as a professional association, the conference approved the first group of four schools for registration, which included two missionary hospital-based schools in Foochow, the Mary Black Hospital of Soochow, and the Shantung Road Hospital of Shanghai. In the following year, the NAC began to hold certification examinations annually. Since practically no standardized textbook for nursing students was available except Hampton-Robb's book, the NAC appealed to the Rockefeller Foundation for funding. In the meantime, Elsie Chung, Gage, and many others translated and introduced some forty books within several years.[34]

The outstanding achievements of the missionary nurses won praise from their missionary colleagues in medicine. In an editorial of its journal in

November 1914 the Medical Missionary Association of China declared, "Nothing in medical mission work in China of the past few years has been more marked in its development than the growth in training schools for both male and female nurses."[35]

Obstacles to Nursing Development

For all its remarkable pace, the incipient development of nursing education was still far behind the rapidly growing demand for nursing personnel. A medical commission sent by the Rockefeller Foundation on a survey tour of China in 1914 reported that there were some 140 foreign nurses in the country distributed in about 100 hospitals. "Less than one hospital in two has a graduate nurse at all."[36]

A number of factors still worked against the development of nursing. One obvious factor, as the report of the Rockefeller Foundation medical commission pointed out, was that "there are few doctors who are qualified to train and supervise nurses."[37] At most nursing schools or hospitals, the task of teaching fell on the shoulders of qualified physicians working in local missionary hospitals. Since missionary doctors were rare and already had their hands full, it was difficult to enlist them for extra work as nursing instructors.

A more fundamental impediment, however, was the scarcity of nursing recruits due to the nation's traditional restrictions on women's social role and their access to education. For centuries, Chinese women, fixed in the role of doing a good job of household work, including bearing and raising the young, had been generally denied the opportunity of getting any schooling. Although Protestant missionaries began to establish boarding schools for girls in the mid-nineteenth century, not until after the 1911 revolution did the republican government recommend for the first time that the lower primary schools be made coeducational and that middle schools for girls be included in the national educational system.[38] The pool of educated Chinese women was therefore very small. Out of this small number, those willing to take nursing for a career constituted an even more insignificant portion.

There were two additional obstacles to women who chose nursing as a career. First, the traditional gender mores prohibited Chinese women from mingling with, still less serving, males they did not know.[39] Respectful of

this tradition, quite a number of hospitals simply separated wards with both patients and nurses by sex. A 1920 survey reported that "up to the present, it is a very great rarity to find female Chinese nurses attending male patients."[40] Second, nursing had never been regarded as a profession in China. Since nursing involved many menial duties, it appeared to be beneath those who had been educated. In spring 1914, Nina Gage reported that two girls at her school had left before the end of the first three months simply because "their families did not wish them to take up nursing."[41] The problem did not disappear quickly. Gage's 1920–1921 report revealed continuous worry over the difficulty of enlisting women with adequate preparation for her school of nursing.[42] To keep students in school, nursing schools adopted the procedure of having students sign contracts. The Hunan-Yale School had the students sign a formal contract requiring them to stay three years after they had successfully gone through the three months' probation. In return, the school committed to teaching them through the three years, providing uniforms and a living stipend.[43] Similar practices were followed at the American Church Mission hospital in Anking and the Temple Hill Hospital, Chefoo, Shantung Province.[44]

Because of the severe shortage of nurses, many institutions, though listed as hospitals, provided practically no nursing at all, the patients being attended by their own friends or servants.[45] At the Lester Chinese Hospital (Shantung Road Hospital) of Shanghai, established by the London Missionary Society in 1843, it was reported that, for all its first-class reputation as one of the oldest hospitals of the city, the hospital had by 1914 only one matron each for its men's and women's sections. When either of the matrons was away or off duty for any reason, the other one had to manage both sections. The institution was thus longing for "more qualified foreign nurses."[46] St. Luke's Hospital, as discussed earlier, had trained two nurses as early as 1887. The early effort had apparently failed, for in 1915, Josiah C. McCracken, dean of the Pennsylvania Medical School of St. John's University, Shanghai, reported vividly to his mission sponsor institution, the Christian Association of the University of Pennsylvania in Philadelphia, of the serious deficiency of nursing at the hospital where his students practiced: "At St. Luke's we have been unusually busy with a good many major operations to do. We do so much need more nursing help. The one foreign nurse that we have is trying to spread herself over the work of four nurses and as a consequence we are not likely to have any nurse long. . . . Nursing at St. Luke's is a hard job for any woman. Nursing at the front would be a picnic compared to it."[47]

Major Developments in the Turbulent Years of the 1920s and 1930s

China entered an age of political turmoil in the mid-1920s when endless strife and fighting tore through the nation. There were wars between regional military leaders, between the revolutionary government in the south and the warlord regime in the north, and later on between the Nationalists and the Communists. To consummate the crisis, the Japanese invaded in the early 1930s. Despite turmoil and chaos, the nursing profession and nursing education underwent, in the words of one missionary nursing leader, a development "unsurpassed in any land at any time in the history of nursing."[48]

The decade of the 1920s began with a landmark event in the history of medicine and nursing in China. Between 1919 and 1921, the Rockefeller Foundation, after years of careful planning and relentless preparation, founded the Peking Union Medical College (PUMC) on the basis of the previous work done by a number of Western missionary organizations in Peking.[49] Intended to be a "Johns Hopkins of the Orient," the PUMC was equipped with the best facilities and a first-class faculty and staff, even by standards of the Western world.[50] The PUMC School of Nursing opened in October 1920. Mandated to give the world's best nursing training, the PUMC nursing school introduced the first joint bachelor of science–Nursing program in China, a venture that preceded many first-rate American nursing schools by two or three decades. Like the PUMC medical school, it required its students to have had two years of preparatory college education, and all the courses were taught in English. Dr. Henry Houghton, PUMC director and dean of the former Harvard Medical School in Shanghai, explicitly expressed his determination to make the nursing profession a "worthy and dignified calling" in order to attract "high class intelligent Chinese Women."[51] Though small in number, the graduates from the PUMC nursing school, mostly appointed to administrative and teaching positions upon graduation, were to play an outstanding role in the future development of nursing in the entire country.[52]

The rapid development of China's nursing in the 1920s can best be seen in the growth of the NAC. From a figure of 132 in 1922, the NAC's membership jumped to around 1,200 in 1926, a ninefold increase in just four years. The schools of nursing registered with the NAC had risen to 112, with a total of 2,000 students enrolled.[53] With the expansion of its scope and resources, the NAC was no longer satisfied with the few pages

the China Medical Missionary Association allowed for its use in the *China Medical Journal*. Beginning in 1920, it published its own quarterly journal, the *Nursing Journal of China,* which carried each article in both English and Chinese. Though small and unostentatious in format, it proved to be vital for academic exchanges among nursing professionals in China.[54]

In order to strengthen its educational activities, the NAC formed the Committee on Nursing Education in 1922. Miss Gage was elected as its chairman and served in that position until her return to the United States in 1927. The committee operated through four subcommittees which were respectively in charge of examinations, translation and publication, curriculum, and registration.[55]

The NAC, which had applied to the International Council of Nurses for membership in 1914, was admitted in 1922, and thus China became the first Asian country to be affiliated with the international nursing society.[56] In 1925, China sent four delegates to the International Council of Nurses Congress in Helsingfors, Finland. Nina Gage was elected the new president of the International Council. The congress also set Peking as the site of its next meeting in 1929.[57]

The spectacular development of nursing in the period can be attributed to two major developments in China — large-scale armed struggle and the rise of nationalism.

Continuous nationwide warfare boosted the number of wounded to be treated. When the Nationalist revolutionary army arrived in Hunan in 1927, wounded soldiers filled the wards, "overflow[ing] every available space" of the missionary hospital in the county of Siangtan.[58] In the heat of a battle between the revolutionary south and the northern warlords in mid-1927, as many as 10,000 wounded soldiers needed emergency treatment. The Red Cross in Shanghai initiated a relief effort for the wounded, calling on medical personnel throughout the country for help. The PUMC, on receiving a request for aid in a personal telegram from Madame Sun Yat-sen, dispatched to Hankow a contingent of eight staff members, among them two missionary nurses and five Chinese nurses. This contingent began its relief work even before the China Medical Board official in charge of the school could have time to clear its involvement with the Rockefeller Foundation headquarters in New York.[59] Ceaseless regional wars brought havoc to large areas and, coupled in many cases with major natural disasters, left thousands of families in dire misery. Mrs. Jean Yates, a graduate of the Roosevelt Hospital Nurses' Training School and a Presbyterian missionary nurse stationed in Hwai Yuan, Anhwei Province, central China, reported in

1932 that in the wake of a flood, the county seat was crowded with refugees and that the women's hospital where she worked "had wards and nurseries crowded beyond capacity."[60]

It was no accident that this era saw a big development of public health nursing in China. In 1925, a district public health station was established in Peking, which gave nurses a major role in administering minimum health care to the public, especially the needy sectors of society. Such a practice for public health care was believed to be the first of its kind not only in China, but in the whole world.[61] Shortly after the Nationalist government formed its Ministry of Health in 1928, the new ministry installed specific agencies to take charge of public health and midwifery.[62] In the early 1930s, along with the shifting of gravity in China's political scene, large-scale experiments got under way to bring health care to China's vast rural areas.

Revolution and nationalism in this turbulent era had a two-pronged impact on the development of nursing in China. First, revolutionary movements, radical or moderate, served to break down old traditions that tended to hold women from playing any active role in society. Stimulated by new revolutionary ideas, more women went to school or tried to win social recognition by taking professional jobs outside their homes. To the new kind of women, nursing provided a good opportunity. The decade of 1926 to 1936 registered a big growth in China's health care. The number of hospitals in China increased from about 100 in 1914 to 500 by 1931. Corresponding to the quick growth of hospitals was an immense development in nursing. By 1936, the NAC membership had jumped to 5,545, representing 174 nursing schools throughout the entire country. In 1936 alone, the NAC granted 638 diplomas to new members.[63] Registered hospital-related schools of nursing were found not only in coastal areas, but in such remote provinces as Hupei, Szechuan, Shansi, Shensi, Kweichow, Liaoning, and Fengtien.[64] Kinwha, a small city in a mountainous area of Chekiang Province, was hardly accessible from outside. Yet a hospital run by the Baptist Mission reported in 1927 that it had a nursing school registered with the NAC. The school, with a student body of sixteen, had doctors and three graduate nurses serving as teachers, and was reportedly producing "good results."[65]

The second effect of the revolutionary movements was the nation's further awakening to its identity among nations. After the Nationalist government settled in Nanking in 1927, the new government established its Ministry of Health in 1928 and advocated a program for a "government system of state medicine." Hospitals and medical and nursing schools were

now required to register with the new ministry. As a result, the pace of nationalization in nursing and health care was quickened. According to a 1932 survey, the proportion of Chinese graduate nurses on nursing staffs throughout China increased from 55 percent in 1920 to 61 percent in 1925 and 74 percent in 1930. The greaesest increase in native nurses was seen in central China, where they increased from 53 percent in 1920 to 78 percent in 1930 (see table 1). In comparison, the increase in the proportion of Chinese doctors was more moderate.[66]

The trend of nationalization can also be seen in the composition of the NAC. In 1922, its members were predominantly Western missionary nurses of diverse nationalities—American, British, Danish, Norwegian, Swedish, Australian. At its annual convention, the official language used was English, and no Chinese person was elected on any committee. By 1926, along with its enormous expansion, Chinese nurses accounted for two-thirds of its membership.[67] For the first time in its short history, the NAC had a large Chinese delegation at its 1926 convention. Chinese was adopted as the official language for the meeting, and Chinese nurses were elected to every committee. One even claimed the office of vice president.[68]

Nationwide turmoil and the process of nationalization in the 1920s and 1930s had a generally unfavorable impact on the Western missions. Willingly or unwillingly, many missionary doctors and nurses quit their positions in China. The Presbyterian South China Mission reported in 1928 that its mission force had been reduced "to a lower figure than for many years."[69] In nursing, Henry S. Houghton, director of the PUMC, observed as early as 1925 that the profession had seen "the greatest progress" in replacement of foreigners by Chinese.[70] In the 1930s, the replacements at the PUMC gradually moved up the ladder to positions of nursing supervisors and instructors. Of the twenty-seven instructors and supervisors appointed during the year 1935 to 1936, thirteen were Chinese nurses.[71] In December 1937, a Chinese nurse graduate was appointed as assistant dean of the School of Nursing. The position was filled in January 1939 by another Chinese graduate, who eventually took over the deanship on Miss Hodgman's departure in 1940.[72] When the school moved to southwest China and reopened in 1943, the teaching staff was composed entirely of its Chinese graduates.[73]

As in the past, revolutionary turmoil and nationalist upsurge landed missionary nurses in the interior provinces in a much worse situation. In many cases, they were confronted with radical masses inflamed with anti-foreign and anti-Christian feelings. The students of a missionary school of

TABLE I.   PERCENTAGE OF CHINESE IN GRADUATE NURSING STAFFS IN 1920, 1925, AND 1930 FOR NORTH, CENTRAL, AND SOUTH CHINA.

Year	North	Central	South	All China
1920	56	53	57	55
1925	57	59	70	61
1930	65	78	75	74

Source: Data from William G. Lennox, "A Self-Survey by Mission Hospitals in China," China Medical Journal 46 (1932): 493–94.

nursing in Hunan Province, for instance, raised sixteen demands to the school authorities. Their first demand was for the school to get registered under the provincial government, which was a direct challenge to the mission's privilege as an independent entity. Other demands included making Bible classes and Sunday services optional, allowing a bigger student voice in school administration, and lightening the workload and study hours ("not to exceed 8 hours daily").[74]

Miss Gage gave a more detailed account of her own experience:

> [E]veryone is unionized now — coolies, servants, clerks, etc., etc. . . . All the rickshas are off the streets nearly every day while parades are going on at the behest of the Union. And then they talk about "Imperialism" . . .
> It seems now just like the old days of the Inquisition and anyone with a grudge whispers it to the Union, or says So and So is anti-revolutionary, and articles come out in the papers, which these days are simply teeming with filth and scurrilous abuse. . . .
> Our servants are all in the union. . . . They demanded more wages, and refuse to let us dismiss anyone and manage with fewer servants than we had. So of course we cannot hold out long, but must go . . . [75]

During the unrest of the 1911 revolution, Miss Gage had taken refuge in Shanghai to wait out the worst months. Fortunately for her, it was not long before she felt that the situation in the province was sufficiently quiet for her return to the nursing school in Changsha. The turmoil in the mid-1920s, however, was so disheartening that she left China for good in 1927.

There are no statistics at hand to show how many missionaries left China in this chaotic period, but when the NAC convened its fourteenth conference in January 1928, its record-high membership of 1,409 included only 400 foreign nurses.[76] The rank of missionary nurses was thus shrinking

in inverse proportion to the quick expansion of Chinese membership in the NAC. At the fifteenth conference in Shanghai two years later, the NAC's membership recorded a new high of 2,000, of which only 200 were missionary nurses.[77] The foreign exodus continued into the 1930s.

The occupation of increasingly larger areas of Chinese territory by the Japanese invaders did not make the life and work of Western missionaries any easier. One missionary nurse named B. Petrie Smith of the Blyth Hospital, English Methodist Mission, who had worked in a medium-sized city called Wenchow in Chekiang Province, had an attack of dysentery during her journey to Shanghai in the summer of 1941. The small coastal steamer she traveled on, unfortunately, was detained by Japanese gunboats. Lacking prompt treatment, she died at a hospital in Shanghai.[78]

Even as they first started their mission in China, missionaries had planned to hand over their work in the future to Chinese health workers when the latter had established a self-sustaining medical profession and administration. One Rockefeller Foundation official asserted in 1915 that the "rapidity" with which the Chinese accepted scientific medicine as their own and the "rapidity" with which the foreign influence diminished "would be the measure of success" for foreign medical enterprises in China.[79] The actual transfer, however, came quicker than missionaries might have expected, and, what is worse, it took a much blunter form than they could have envisioned. In the stormy years of 1927 and 1928, the Commission of China of the Protestant Episcopal Church in the United States blamed the "agitation for control" of mission property in China on "a few extremists whose enthusiasm outruns their judgment and who overestimate their ability to administer trusts properly." The church contended that such a forced and premature transfer would "undo the work of years" by the missionaries and harm China. While asserting that "no transfer of any description can be entertained," the church nevertheless resigned itself to the prospect of shifting funds from China to its mission work elsewhere.[80]

Summary

By the late 1930s, nursing, which had come into being in China in the 1880s, had developed into a profession represented by a well-organized national association with a membership of 6,000, which was continuously expanding by hundreds of new recruits trained at nearly 200 nursing schools all over the country. The progress was remarkable. In retrospect, we can

easily discern the outstanding contribution made by the Western medical missionaries. To the latter's dedication, the profession owed its birth and its incipient growth in particular. Trained missionary nurses, following in the footsteps of missionary pioneers, penetrated into all parts of the country to start dispensaries and hospitals literally from nothing. In 1923, China had 53 percent of the missionary hospital beds and 48 percent of the missionary doctors in the world. Missionary nurses constituted 32 percent of the total number of nurses in China in 1923 and their number reached a peak of nearly 700 in 1927.[81] Although the number of medical missionaries, physicians, and nurses was tiny compared to the size of the nation's population, and although their interest in "healing the sick" aimed to serve their primary goal of "saving the soul," their contribution to nursing development in China, especially their efforts in training native nurses at numerous missionary hospitals and nursing schools, can hardly be overestimated.

Derived from missionary involvement was another important contributor to the rapid progress of nursing: the Nurses' Association of China. Born in a critical stage of nursing development in the country, the NAC organized the profession and regulated its training through sponsoring registration, holding examinations, and developing a standard required curriculum. Essentially, it played the role of a great organizer and paved the way for the further growth of the profession.

Coming from a totally different culture, missionaries had to overcome a lot of difficulty to adapt themselves to the environment in China. The problems they encountered varied from place to place. Geographically, the interior areas were more prone to antiforeign and anti-Christian feelings, whereas the coastal areas were, comparatively, more receptive to new ideas and techniques brought by Western missionaries. Fluctuating with the political developments in China, the missionaries' cause peaked when the nation welcomed them following the quelling of the Boxer upheaval and the overthrow of the dynastic monarchy, and ebbed when xenophobia or nationalism ran high in any form of massive political turmoil. Notwithstanding political problems, each missionary's success or failure depended very much on the individual's ability to accommodate the native culture and society.

As many authors have pointed out, the work of missionaries contributed not only to the propagation of new techniques and knowledge in China, but, indirectly, to the awakening of the sense of democracy in the population.[82] In nursing, the living role models of female missionary nurses working confidently and unrestrainedly side by side with male physicians

enlightened the minds of many Chinese regarding the irrationality of the nation's age-old traditions of social gender segregation.[83] As one revolutionary movement after another destroyed old traditions and released women from ancient cultural bondages, the ranks of nursing swelled with increasingly large numbers of new recruits. Although not yet full-fledged in expertise and lacking especially in administrative experience, the Chinese nurses won recognition as a new and independent professional force in the turbulent decade of the 1930s.

Paradoxically, through introducing new knowledge and values into the country, the missionaries indirectly cultivated the mounting revolutionary movements that would make their work increasingly difficult. Japan's invasion further complicated the missions' situation. Missionary nurses left the country at a speed exceeding what would have been desirable for a sound consolidation of the new profession. Finally, when the Communists took over the country in 1949, all the missions were forced to withdraw from China. Although their work was thus terminated, the missionaries left behind a rich legacy through their work in such secular fields as medicine, nursing, health care, education, and charity. Their help with the development of nursing in China for over half a century forms a fascinating chapter in the history of the nation's health care as well as in the history of international cultural exchanges.

KAIYI CHEN, PHD
University Archives
North Arcade, Franklin Field
University of Pennsylvania
Philadelphia, PA 19104-6320
Phone: (215) 898-7024

Notes

1. See Anna C. Jamme, "Nursing Education in China," *American Journal of Nursing* 23 (1923): 666–67 (hereafter cited as *AJN*); Xu-dong Zhu, "Review of the Development of Nursing in China," *Nursing Journal of China* 17, no. 4 (1936); K. Chimin Wong and Lien-teh Wu, *History of Chinese Medicine* (Shanghai: National Quarantine Service, 1936), 449, 453.

2. See Jamme; Xu-dong Zhu; and Wong and Wu, 449, 453.

3. The Woman's Hospital of Philadelphia Records, the Center for the Study of the History of Nursing, University of Pennsylvania.

4. "List of Medical Missionaries in China, Corea and Siam," *China Medical Missionary Journal* 1 (1887): 34–37. The *China Medical Missionary Journal* (hereaf-

ter cited as *CMMJ*) was the official journal of the Medical Missionary Association of China. It changed its name in 1907 to *China Medical Journal* (hereafter cited as *CMJ*).

    5. "Introductory," *CMMJ* (1887): 29–30.

    6. H. W. Boone, "The Medical Missionary Association of China — Its Future Work," *CMMJ* 1 (1887): 1–8.

    7. *Chinese Recorder* 18 (1887): 42.

    8. See Second Annual Report of the Philander Smith Memorial Hospital, Nanking, *CMMJ* 3 (1889): 29–30; and Wong and Wu, 486.

    9. Wong and Wu, 486, 529.

    10. See "Instruction of Native Students" and "Hospital Reports," *CMMJ* 10 (1896): 162 and 271.

    11. "President's Address," *CMMJ* 3 (1889): 109–14.

    12. Jane Hunter, "Domestic Empire" in *The Gospel of Gentility: American Women Missionaries in Turn-of-the Century China* (New Haven, Conn.: Yale University Press, 1984), 128–73.

    13. See G. H. Choa, *"Heal the Sick" Was Their Motto: The Protestant Medical Missionaries in China* (Hong Kong: The Chinese University Press, 1990), 190–191; and Jessie Gregory Lutz, *China and the Christian Colleges, 1850–1985* (Ithaca, N.Y.: Cornell University Press, 1971), 7–11.

    14. Peter Kong-ming New and Yuet-wah Cheung, "Early Years of Medical Missionary Work in the Canadian Presbyterian Mission in North Honan, China, 1887–1900: Healing the Heathens and the Missionaries," *Asian Profile* 12, no. 5 (October 1984). See also *CMMJ* 14 (1900): 296–302; and *CMMJ* 15 (1901): 81–82.

    15. See *CMMJ* 20 (1906): 188–89; and *CMJ* 23 (1909): 344–45.

    16. Wong and Wu, 557.

    17. See *CMJ* 23 (1909): 119–20, 342–43; and *CMJ* 26 (1912): 190.

    18. "Temple Hill Hospital, American Presbyterian Mission, Chefoo, China, Report, 1917," Presbyterian Historical Society.

    19. "Presbyterian Mission Hospital (South), Soochow, 1915–1916," Rockefeller Archive Center, RG 4, series 1, box 22, folder 445 (hereafter cited as RAC).

    20. Harriet M. Allyn to Arthur Brown, 23 August 1915, Presbyterian Historical Society, RG 82 (China Mission), box 1, folder 18: "Canton — Correspondence re Medical Situation, 1909–1925."

    21. See Mary H. Fulton, *Twenty-Five Years of Medical Work in China* (Philadelphia: The Women's Foreign Missionary Society of the Presbyterian Church, 1909); M. Adelaide Nutting, *A History of Nursing*, vol. 4 (New York: G. P. Putnam's Sons, 1907–1912), 279–280; and *CMJ* 23 (1909): 121.

    22. See *The Canton Christian College Newsletter*, no. 11, 7 July 1913, Information Files, University Archives, University of Pennsylvania (hereafter cited as Penn Archives); and William W. Cadbury to Board of Directors of the University Medical School in Canton, 1 September 1914, Christian Assoc. Rec., Committee Series, Penn Archives; and "Report of Work Done by W. W. Cadbury During Eight Months at the Kung Ye Hospital," Christian Assoc. Rec., Committee Series, Penn Archives.

23. See William W. Cadbury to Marshall S. Morgan, 26 May 1913, Christian Assoc. Rec., Committee Series, Penn Archives; *The Canton Christian College Newsletter*, No. 11 (7 July 1913), Information Files, Penn Archives; News clipping, *Bulletin* (Philadelphia), 20 October 1910, Information Files, Penn Archives; and *Old Penn,* vol. XI, no. 8 (16 November 1912), Information Files, Penn Archives.

24. Wong and Wu, 557.

25. See *AJN* 8 (December 1907): 189; and *AJN* 9 (March 1909): 424–26, 584–85.

26. Wong and Wu, 557.

27. See Minutes, Annual Reports—Proceedings of Executive Committee, 1901–1909, Yale-in-China Collection, Sterling Memorial Library, Yale University, series I, box 1; "Yale-in-China Annual Reports, 1909–1912," box 11, folder 96; and "Report of the Governing Board, April 1914," box 11, folder 97: "Annual Reports of the Department of the College of Yale in China, 1913–1916," Yale-in-China Collection.

28. "Yale in China, Annual reports, 1909–1912," Yale-in-China Collection.

29. See Minutes, Annual Reports—Proceedings of Executive Committee, 1901–1901, Yale-in-China Collection; "Yale-in-China Annual Reports, 1909–1912"; and "Report of the Governing Board, April 1914."

30. *CMJ* 20 (1906): 86.

31. Constitution of the Nurses' Association of China, *CMJ* 24 (1910): 81.

32. See Nina D. Gage, "Life at Yali," January 1930, Yale-in-China Collection, box 66, folder 204; and Wong and Wu, 560–62.

33. Gage, "Life in Yali."

34. See Gage, "Life in Yali"; Wong and Wu, 560–62; and Cora E. Simpson, *A Joy Ride Through China for the N.C.A.* (Shanghai: Kwang Hsueh Publishing House, 1922), 15.

35. *CMJ* 28 (November 1914): 406.

36. Announcement of the Rockefeller Foundation, 7 March 1915, RAC, Rockefeller Foundation, RG 4, box 10, folder 131, "Mission Societies, 1914–1918."

37. Roger S. Greene, "Medical Needs of the Chinese," reprint from *The Chinese Recorder,* April 1918, Christian Assoc. Rec., Committee Series, box 4, folder 55, Penn Archives.

38. See Ping-wen Kao, *The Chinese System of Public Education* (New York: Teachers College, Columbia University, 1915), 101, 111, 121, 129; and Lutz, 131.

39. Hunter, 21–22.

40. Harold Balme and Milton T. Stauffer, "An Enquiry into the Scientific Efficiency of Mission Hospitals in China," presented at the Annual Conference of the China Medical Missionary Association, 21–27 February 1920, Peking, China, Presbyterian Historical Society.

41. Nina D. Gage, "Report of the Training School for Nurses, 1914," Yale-in-China Collection, box 11, folder 97.

42. Nina D. Gage, "Report of the Human-Yale School of Nursing, 1 June 1920 to 31 May 1921," Yale-in-China Collection, box 44, folder 444.

43. Gage, "Life in Yali."

44. See *CMJ* 23 (1909): 344; and "Temple Hill Hospital, American Presbyte-

rian Mission, Chefoo, China, Report, 1917," Presbyterian Historical Society, Shantung Mission File.

45. Greene, "Medical Needs of the Chinese."

46. "Shantung Road Hospital, Shanghai, 1914," RAC, Rockefeller Foundation, RG 4, China Medical Board, series 1, box 22, folder 438. According to M. Adelaide Nutting, an Australian nurse, Sister Ethel Halley went to work at the Shantung Road Hospital in Shanghai in 1890 or 1891. Sister Halley later recollected that
she had worked in China for 15 years before she had any Chinese nurses work with
her (Nutting, 277).

47. Josiah McCracken to Edward C. Wood, 8 May 1915, Christian Assoc.
Rec., Committee Series, Penn Archives.

48. Cora E. Simpson, "With Our Nurses," *Chinese Recorder* 56 (1925): 22–25.

49. The precursor of the PUMC was the Union Medical College, a joint enterprise of a group of Western church organizations, among them the London Missionary Society, the London Medical Missionary Association, the American Presbyterian Missionary Society, the Methodist Missionary Society, and the American
Board of Missions (Congregational). See Mary Ferguson, *China Medical Board and
Peking Union Medical College* (New York: China Medical Board of New York,
1970), 20 and footnote.

50. Modeled after the German pattern of medical education, Johns Hopkins
University was the first American university that required a four-year liberal arts
college education before admittance to the medical school. The university was also
noted for laying emphasis on research and laboratory work and introducing the
concept of medical science into medical education. The Rockefeller Foundation
leaders wanted to introduce this model to China. See Mary Brown Bullock, "A
Johns Hopkins for China," in *An American Transplant: The Rockefeller Foundation
and Peking Union Medical College* (Berkeley: University of California Press, 1980),
24–27.

51. Henry S. Houghton to Dr. McLean, 26 April 1918, RAC, China Medical
Board of New York Archives (hereafter cited as CMB), RG IV 2 B 9, box 98, folder
704: "Nurses, 1918–1926."

52. I intend to discuss in a separate paper PUMC's contribution to nursing
development in China.

53. "On the Field," *Chinese Recorder* 57 (1926): 303.

54. See Gage, "Life in Yali"; and Wong and Wu, 560–62.

55. Gage, "Life in Yali."

56. Ibid.

57. "On the Field," 224. Due to the developments in China, the meeting place
of the next International Congress of Nurses was later changed.

58. "Report of E. D. Vanderburgh, 1926–1927," Presbyterian Historical Society, RG 82, box 34, folder 1: "Reports, 1927."

59. See H. S. Houghton, interview with H. V. A. MacMurray, American minister, 2 June 1927, RAC, CMB, box 125, folder 904; and cables between PUMC staff
and CMB in New York, RAC, Rockefeller Foundation, RG 4, series 2, box 65,
folders 1613 and 1614, box 50, folder 1153.

60. Hospital sketch of the Cragin Memorial Hospital for Women and Chi'-

dren, Presbyterian Historical Society, Yates Family Papers, box 3, folder: "Miscellaneous Reports, 1922–1981."

61. See Gertrude E. Hodgman, "PUMC School of Nursing, 1931," CMB, box 98, folder 706; Mary Ferguson, *China Medical Board and Peking Union Medical College,* 57–58; and Bullock, 95.

62. Wong and Wu, 719–21.

63. See the 13th Biennial Conference of the Nurses' Association of China, Nanking, October 1936, *Nursing Journal of China* 18 (January 1937); and list of schools of nursing registered with the Nurses' Association of China, *Nursing Journal of China* 18 (January 1937): appendix.

64. Membership roll up to 1 July 1936, *Nursing Journal of China* 18 (1937).

65. Wong Chen-hao, "The Indigenous Church Movement in Kinhwa," *Chinese Recorder* 58 (1927): 35–39.

66. William G. Lennox, "A Self Survey by Mission Hospitals in China," *CMJ,* 46 (1932): 493–94.

67. Another source put the figure of Chinese nurses for the beginning of 1925 at 561 (350 female, 211 male). See L. C. Goodrich to Roger S. Greene, 12 February 1925, RAC, CMB, RG IV 2 B 9, box 107, folder 711: "Nurses Association of China, 1925–1946."

68. Cora E. Simpson to R. S. Greene, 16 December 1926, RAC, Rockefeller Foundation, RG 4, series 1, box 64, folder 1577.

69. "South China Mission, 1928," Presbyterian Historical Society, RG 82, box 35, folder 18: "Minutes and Reports, 1928."

70. See Henry S. Houghton, "The Director's Report, 1924–1925," RAC, CMB, RG IV 2 B 9, box 98, folder 704; Roger S. Greene, interview with Miss R. Ingram, 26 August 1927, RAC, CMB RG IV 2 B 9, box 98, folder 705; and Henry S. Houghton to M. K. Eggleton, 1 November 1927, with minutes of the Hospital Committee meeting of 28 October 1927 attached, RAC, CMB RG IV 2 B 9, box 98, folder 705.

71. Faculty and Nursing Staff, 1935–1936, RAC, CMB, RG IV 2 B 9, box 99, folder 710.

72. Governing Council—Educational Division, 4 December 1937, RAC, CMB, RG IV 2 B 9, box 99, folder 707; H. S. Houghton to E. C. Lobenstine, 9 December 1938, RAC, CMB RG IV 2 B 9.

73. "Alumnae News," no. IX, RAC, CMB, box 99, folder 711.

74. "Sixteen Demands by Students of the P'u Chi School of Nursing, Yochow, Hunan," RAC, CMB, box 98, folder 705.

75. Nina D. Gage to Mr. Bevis, 12 December 1926, Yale-in-China Collection, box 66, folder 209.

76. Ruth Ingram, diary of her attendance at the conference of the NAC, January 1928, RAC, CMB, box 98, folder 705. According to K. Chimin Wong, the number of missionary nurses was about 700 in 1927. (See Wong and Wu, 562.)

77. Wong and Wu, 562. According to the Prayer List of 1931, the total number of foreign nurses in that year was 256. (See Lennox, 484–534).

78. "In Remembrance," *Chinese Recorder* 72 (1941): 35.

79. W. H. Welch, address to members of the Saturday Club, Shanghai,

30 October 1915, RAC, Rockefeller Foundation, History Source Material, vol. 3, 587.

80. "Protestant Episcopal Church in the U.S.A., Division of Missions, Report of the Commission to China, October 1927–March 1928," Presbyterian Historical Society.

81. See Lennox, 484–534; and Wong and Wu, 562.

82. See Lutz, 526, 528–29; Hunter, 179–81; Choa, 205; and John K. Fairbank, ed., *The Missionary Enterprise in China and America* (Cambridge, Mass.: Harvard University Press, 1974), 3, 12–14.

83. Hunter, 26, 181, 263–64.

Agnes Karll and the Creation of an Independent German Nursing Association, 1900–1927

GEERTJE BOSCHMA
School of Nursing
University of Pennsylvania

Nursing in Late-Nineteenth-Century Germany

Nursing turmoil in late-nineteenth-century Germany was signaled by strikes of dissatisfied deaconess nurses and sisters of the order of St. John in some of the hospitals in Hamburg.[1] Not only was inappropriate care in the hospitals widely discussed in the newspapers, but influential physicians, members of parliament, and practicing nurses themselves began to question the lack of legal regulations and proper education for nurses. While some people blamed nurses for being uncivilized and uneducated, others argued that nurses were victims of exploitation and inappropriate labor conditions.[2]

The provocative publication "Die soziale Stellung der Krankenpfleger-innen" (The Social Position of Nurses) by Elisabeth Storp, a nurse trained in the Victoria House in Berlin, stirred public debate. Storp discussed the working conditions and exploitation of German nurses and compared the wages of nurses with those of teachers. Storp challenged nurses to establish a committee to advocate state-approved education and legal protection of nurses' work.[3] Her agenda reflected that of the growing women's movement and women's concomitant desire for professional respect and public rights.

This "revolt against unpaid labor of women"[4] reflects a period of nursing's transition from a charitable and religious enterprise to a paid professional occupation.[5] At the beginning of the nineteenth century, university-educated physicians gradually gained dominance and sought educated assistants who could follow their orders. However, their efforts to improve

Nursing History Review 4 (1996): 151–68. Copyright © 1996 by The American Association for the History of Nursing.

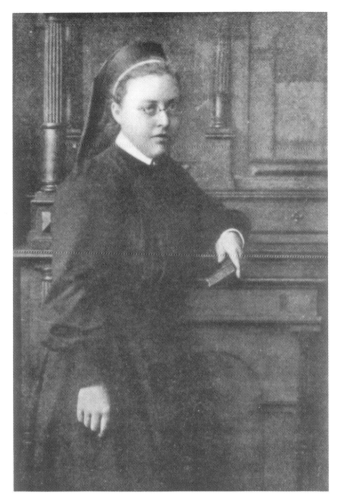

Figure 1. Sister Agnes Karll.

hospital nursing care by introducing training for attendants and nurses had had only limited effect. Though physicians established a six-month training course in the Berliner Charité hospital in 1832, the training was narrowly focused on medical matters and did not change the poor working conditions under which nurses practiced. Thus, since middle- and upper-class women were reluctant to practice in hospitals, the work continued to attract primarily laborers of society's lower class.[6]

The dominant organizations nursing the sick during the nineteenth century were religious or charitable nursing orders. Catholic orders had flourished since early in the century. Protestants seeking involvement in the care of the sick followed the example of the Catholic orders by reviving the function of the deaconess. The most famous deaconess institute was in Kaiserswerth, established by Pastor Theodor Fliedner in 1836.[7] Motivated by missionary zeal, Fliedner undertook many social reforms. By 1850 the Kaiserswerth Institute consisted of "a hospital nursing school, a mother-house [for nurses and teachers], an orphanage, a teachers seminary for infant, elementary and industrial schoolteachers, an infant school and an asylum for the female mentally ill."[8]

Catholic sisters and Protestant deaconesses were organized in mother-houses. Within the motherhouse structure, women from respected families were able to pursue a socially accepted public role. Devoting themselves to works of charity, sisters were bound to the motherhouse for life. In exchange for their work, they received shelter, food, clothing, pocket money, and provisions for old age.[9] The sisters did not receive any personal salary. The structure of the motherhouse was strictly hierarchical; sisters went wherever the head of the house sent them. Often sisters or deaconesses took over the entire care and management of hospitals with which the order contracted.

Nurse training in the motherhouses was grounded in the principles of order, discipline, and obedience, and it generally contained some medical instruction.[10] Fliedner emphasized the role of women in the care of the sick and designed a detailed rule of conduct for the deaconess sisterhood in order to make nursing an acceptable career for middle-class women. The motherhouse system was such a powerful model that even patriotic associations for the care of wounded soldiers, established during the nineteenth century and eventually merging into the Red Cross organization, imitated the motherhouse idea.[11]

By the end of the nineteenth century, sociopolitical, economic, and cultural changes increased the demand for nurses. By 1900, rapid industrialization propelled Germany into one of the largest industrial powers of Europe.[12] The population increased from forty million in 1870 to forty-nine and a half million in 1890, and to almost sixty-eight million in 1914, generating a major migration to urban and industrial areas. Population growth, the development of a growing industrial proletariat, and a rising middle class dramatically changed the health needs of the people and increased the need for nurses both in hospitals and private homes. The 1848 epidemics of

typhus and cholera, hitting hardest among the poor, had shown revolutionary physicians such as Rudolf Virchow the relationship between poverty,
social and economic living conditions, and health.[13] Gradually, these physicians' ideas on social responsibility and health promotion for the working
poor disseminated and appeared in various initiatives of preventive medicine during the late nineteenth and early twentieth centuries.

Initiated as a nursing reform at the beginning of the nineteenth century, the motherhouse system turned out to be too rigid and inflexible by
the end of the century. In the rapidly growing cities, many nurses separated
themselves from the motherhouses and began to work either in private duty
or in the municipal hospitals. Changing views about women's role in society, a growing women's movement, and the need for women to make a
living fostered the idea among many nurses that the motherhouses were too
restrictive. Like women in general, a new generation of nurses sought economic independence and an autonomous life.[14]

However, the "free" or "wild" nurses, as those who had separated
themselves from motherhouses were called,[15] were still vulnerable, risking
their reputations and remaining largely unprotected and isolated. Accepting pay for service provided an opportunity to earn a living, but work
conditions, especially in the urban hospitals, were harsh. Subsidized by
charity and endowments, motherhouses could provide service for prices
that were far lower than those of self-supporting nurses. To compete with
motherhouses, they had to accept low wages and poor working conditions.[16] Even motherhouses often depleted their resources to support old
and disabled sisters.[17] Nurses were not included in state social security laws
for sickness, disability, and old age. Unfortunately, many experienced poor
physical or mental health at early ages.[18] Lack of legal protection or regulation of training for nurses made independent nurses prone to exploitation.

Agnes Karll

It was exactly this situation that Agnes Karll planned to change when she
founded the Professional Organization for German Nurses (POGN) in
1903.[19] Agnes Karll (1868–1927),[20] daughter of an estate owner, initially
attended a preparatory school for teachers,[21] but then decided to enter
nurse training. At age nineteen, she entered the Clementinen House in
Hannover, a Red Cross motherhouse. Eventually, family obligations forced
Karll to perform independent work and she worked in private duty in Ber-

lin from 1891 to 1901.[22] Though her cases were primarily from higher social classes and referred from a group of well-educated family doctors,[23] the work culminated in her physical breakdown at age thirty-three (1901).[24]

The year 1901 was a turning point in Agnes Karll's life. As her over-strained and weakened physical condition forced her to abandon private duty, she devoted herself to the betterment of nurses' social and working conditions. Her own personal experiences gave her a clear understanding of the needs of nurses and the courage and commitment to act as a leader.[25]

Though Karll did not yet have a clear idea of how she would pursue her ideals for nursing improvement, she used two important resources to develop her ideas: her connections with the women's movement and her knowledge about insurance opportunities for nurses. During her years in private duty, friends had kept her up to date on the literature on women's affairs, even though she had not actively participated in the women's movement.[26] She had also looked into state and private insurance opportunities for nurses, searching for solutions to how nurses could protect themselves financially for the risk of old age and disability.[27] These sources helped her conceptualize something new and look for people and organizations who could assist her to realize her plans for improving the condition of nurses.

During this period, Karll became acquainted with Adele Schreiber, one of the first women appointed by a private insurance company, the Duetsche Anker, to look after the insurance needs of a growing group of employed women.[28] Compulsory social insurance for laborers had been implemented in Germany by state law in the late nineteenth century.[29] However, as noted earlier, nurses were not included in the state insurance program.[30] Schreiber helped Karll envision a strategy for providing nurses with private insurance. As a result of this relationship, Karll became the first nurse insured with the Deutsche Anker. Schreiber introduced Karll to the director, who demonstrated an interest in the cause of nurses.[31] Moreover, he supported Karll in her idea to create a nurses' association in an effort to improve nurses' socioeconomic welfare. He welcomed the opportunity to provide private insurance for nurses. The Deutsche Anker remained very supportive of Karll. It may be speculated that Karll's subsequent part-time position with an unnamed insurance company after her illness may well have been with this company.[32]

At this time, Karll became interested in the publications of Elisabeth Storp and Marie Cauer. Cauer, a nurse writing about the condition of nurses, was the stepdaughter of a leading figure in the German women's movement.[33] During the summer of 1902, Karll met with Storp, Cauer, and

Cauer's associate, Helene Meyer, in Berlin.[34] The professional plight of nurses had attracted the attention of the League of German Women's Associations (GWA) through Storp's brochure.[35] At the time, the GWA not only supported suffrage as a way to promote women's role in public life, it also advocated women's right to work and to attain higher education.[36] The GWA's leaders agreed to accept a paper on nursing at the 1902 national meeting of the association in Wiesbaden; Cauer, Karll, Storp, and Meyer were invited to prepare and present the paper.

Initially, Karll was hesitant about participating in this group, since her primary interest lay in improving the situation of independent private duty nurses. The others were more concerned with changing the training and working conditions for hospital-based nurses through licensing and state registration. Despite a seeming conflict of interest, however, discussions among the other nurses and the leaders of the GWA about self-organization convinced Karll to participate.[37] Gradually, Karll began to see the need for self-organization and the improvement of education and legal regulation as two complementary strategies toward the achievement of nurses' social improvement.

While preparing for the Wiesbaden meeting, Cauer, Karll, Storp, and Meyer found further support from theology professor Dr. Friedrich Zimmer, the founder of the Evangelical Deaconess Association,[38] established in 1894. Zimmer's Association differed from the traditional Fliedner-type motherhouse system. Zimmer attracted middle- and upper-class women wanting to do professional work in a paid position.[39] Although he received criticism from the motherhouses who perceived service for pay inconsistent with deaconess work, Zimmer viewed his effort as the evangelical church's contribution to the resolution of the women's question. He supported the women's movement and especially nurses' aspiration to state exams and registration.[40]

The Wiesbaden meeting was Karll's first public event. The Deutsche Anker supported her initiative and paid for her travel expenses.[41] Participating in the meeting with 230 other women, Karll was immediately caught up in the excitement of great gatherings of women.[42] This meeting strongly supported the idea of professional independence for nurses. During the meeting, Karll made valuable contacts and was encouraged by other participants to seek some form of self-organization for nurses.[43] The paper presented by Cauer, Karll, Storp, and Meyer clearly outlined the need for state protection of nurse training, with subsequent registration, as well as the need to improve nurses' labor conditions.[44] The meeting made it clear to

Karll that some form of self-organization was imperative for independent nurses; the GWA provided the model for putting the plan into action.

The POGN and Its Nursing Bureau

The strong support for her ideas at Wiesbaden provided the impetus for Karll to implement her work immediately. Back in Berlin, she took to heart the advice to fight for the goals of independent nurses through self-organization. Ironically, Karll thought that such an organization could not be successfully created without the support of men.[45] Hitherto all nursing associations had adopted the motherhouse model, which was always headed by a man. She approached two medical officials, asking them to act as organization president and treasurer.[46] Both men were supportive; in fact, they encouraged Karll to seek nurses to sit on the board of the professional organization. Nurses themselves, they believed, were best able to judge professional nursing matters.

Karll gathered a group of seven nurses to form the preparatory committee for the foundation of an independent organization for nurses, the POGN. After studying American examples, Karll designed a draft of the organization's bylaws with the help of Maria Cauer.[47] The objective was to form an organization that actively mediated private duty nurses' placement through an employment bureau. Those who hired the nurses would have to pay them their salary directly. This was quite a change from the motherhouse system, in which the association received the pay and the nurses obtained some pocket money. The bylaws also required that members of the organization seek some form of financial protection for illness and old age through insurance.[48]

Along with providing socioeconomic support, the POGN would create a forum to represent the independent nurses in the political realm. It sought to improve the status of nursing through advocating state regulation of nurse training and regulation of labor conditions. Through a journal, regular meetings, and lectures, the members would keep in contact and make their voice heard publicly.

A founding meeting held on 11 January 1903 attracted about thirty nurses. These nurses, the first members of the organization, elected the preparatory committee as the board of directors and Agnes Karll as the POGN's president. Because most of the women were unfamiliar with leadership responsibilities, they were hesitant to take responsibility for secre-

tarial and managerial tasks. Karll noted that "none of us had ever taken minutes, not to mention ever having chaired a meeting."[49] The operation of running a business was a new experience for women in general; much of what the nurses learned was through trial and error. Each step, Karll noted, had to be thought through, planned, and tried. Karll and her group of colleagues gave all their spare time and energy to the establishment of the POGN and the nursing bureau. Initially the bureau had one paid worker. In order to be recognized as a legal body, the POGN had to obtain corporation rights from local governmental officials. The bylaws were printed and sent to 2,400 physicians in Berlin and its suburbs.[50] Within a year, the POGN had 300 members.

Karll became a strong advocate of nurses' insistence on keeping the control of their work in their own hands.[51] An extensive network was created among nurses throughout the country, and various local subdivisions were established, headed by a nurse if at all possible. Karll traveled extensively, speaking to nurses, city officials, women, and physicians about the new idea of an independent nursing association. By the end of the first decade of the twentieth century, the POGN was a flourishing organization with over 3,000 members. The POGN established its own journal in 1905, for which Karll wrote most of the editorials. During the first five years, the bureau grew into a busy office with about ten paid workers.

The POGN had a tense relationship with the motherhouses and many other traditional associations, which felt threatened by the new independent organization. When the POGN chose the Lazarus Cross as their badge, a sign once carried by a knightly order during the crusades, the Red Cross motherhouses complained that the symbol was too close to that of the Red Cross. The POGN won the lawsuit that the Red Cross initiated.[52] Moreover, during their first public meeting, POGN nurses were challenged by some influential physicians because they called themselves "sisters." The use of this title, which expressed public respect for the work of the nurse, was defended by one of the board members, who argued that independent professional nurses were forming a sisterhood as well. The goals of service of a professional organization could only be reached through sisterly unity.[53]

The POGN received major support from the Deutsche Anker. The company paid for Karll's first trips to establish the local divisions. It also provided a special insurance policy for POGN members. The Deutsche Anker paid the POGN 3 percent of the insurance fee for every POGN nurse who took a policy with them. The company also deposited 10 percent of the first insurance fee in the support fund created by the POGN for impe-

cunious members. Karll always stressed the importance of insurance for nurses. Women, she argued, were not yet used to thinking about financial protection.[54] Although POGN members were not obligated to be policy-holders of Deutsche Anker insurance, they had to seek some form of insurance.

Karll kept in close contact with the local groups and maintained strong personal interest in each of the POGN nurses. Lavinia Dock described Karll as a woman with "dominating strength and intense energy, [whose] loving kindness and compassion [were directed by] an intellect keen, search-ing and forceful."[55] Karll was very devoted to the "weal and woe" of the nurses.[56] As the POGN expanded, she actively mediated the placement of nurses not only in private duty but also in hospitals.[57] One of her main concerns was the poor health and relatively high suicide rate among nurses. She sent many personal letters to express her sorrow over the plight of nurses. In a letter to Lavinia Dock, Karll wrote, "Saturday I have to go to a little town one hour distant to look after one of our sisters, who tried to take her life, because she feels, she will not very long be able to work. It is heart rending."[58]

Another way Karll sought to improve the situation of nurses was to show empirical evidence of their current situation. Karll insisted on gather-ing statistics about the condition of the members. In all likelihood, her experience at the insurance office supported her view that statistics were an important tool in publicizing the tragedy of nursing's living and working conditions, demonstrating the need for reform. Karll developed an exten-sive demographic questionnaire for all POGN members, which included questions about age, previous positions, age of entry in nursing, length of nursing practice, membership in federations/motherhouses, history of ill-ness, working hours, hours and days off, holidays, hours and frequency of nightshifts, wages, care in case of sickness or disability, old age, causes of death, and age and annuity at death.[59] So serious was Karll to ascertain statistical data that nurses could be refused membership if they did not fill out the form. Karll gathered 2,500 forms by the end of 1909, and from then on each new applicant had to complete the questionnaire.

The International Connections of the POGN

Probably through connections with the international women's movement, Karll's efforts attracted the attention of international nursing leaders who had organized themselves into the International Council of Nurses (ICN)

in 1899. In 1904, the ICN invited Karll to speak at the meeting of the International Council of Women in Berlin.[60] During the meeting, the POGN was accepted as the national German nurses' association.

The connection with international colleagues was valuable to Karll. She envied the accomplishments of American and English colleagues and thought that the unity of the American and English nursing organizations contrasted greatly with the narrow-minded "caste" mentality of the German nursing leaders.[61] Contacts with the international leaders were not only an important intellectual resource but also a strong support for Karll's ideas on independence for nurses through self-organization. Karll kept regular correspondence with Lavinia Dock, with whom she shared both her hopes and frustrations concerning German nursing developments.[62]

The model of nurse training Karll promoted was in accordance with ICN standards. She advocated a state-regulated three-year training program. The eventual outcome of the German political battle over nursing education was disappointing for Karll. Zimmer, who had been invited by the Prussian state government to write a report on the organization of nursing, proposed a state examination after one year of proper training. This became the design for the state registration of nurses effective in Prussia in 1907 and soon after that in many other states.[63] Although Karll was optimistic that the law was an important first step, she was frustrated that nurses had little if any control over the content of the examination. Physicians examined the nurses, and hospital nurse superintendents were unable to voice their opinion about the nurse examinees' success or failure.[64]

Karll's leadership was very much appreciated among the international nurses. At the 1909 ICN meeting in London, Karll was elected ICN president. She served as president until 1912, when the fourth international meeting of the ICN was held in Cologne. Many presentations were given on the social conditions of nurses. The medical official Dr. H. Hecker gave an influential presentation on the overstrain of nurses.

Karll strongly encouraged POGN nurses to attend international meetings. She considered organizations such as the POGN to be a valuable link with larger national and international bodies and an avenue to social progress. Moreover, she saw the linkage of the POGN with the women's movement and the ICN as crucial for the POGN's contribution to the betterment of humankind. How forceful the American example was to Karll is evidenced by her efforts to establish an advanced education program for graduate nurses. Using the Teachers College Nursing Department at Columbia University as a prototype, Karll helped to establish a two-year pro-

gram for advanced nursing education for heads of nursing schools at the School for Higher Education for Women in Leipzig (1912). The program existed only briefly, however, due to the outbreak of the First World War in 1914.[65]

Notwithstanding Karll's appreciation of the ICN relationship, some of its policies disappointed her. The domination of the Anglo-American leaders and Karll's idea that German nursing had not reached their level prevented her from expressing her sometimes different view too strongly among her ICN friends. One of the sources of her frustration was the ICN rule that only nurses graduated from a three-year general hospital course could become active members of the ICN. Because of this restriction, a whole group of influential and highly respected nurses were denied direct membership. Within the context of national public health policy, German health officers had developed a separate training system for preventive health workers and social nurses.[66] They had their own professional organization, although the POGN accepted them as members. Furthermore, after the First World War, specialized training courses were set up for mother and infant care. Nurses who enrolled in this training received a separate diploma for the nursing of children. It was these specialized nurses, who, although considered similar to hospital nurses, were unable to become full members of the international body. To Karll's chagrin, the only thing she could do was to change the name of the POGN to "Professional Organization for Nurses, Nurses of Children and Social Nurses," which was approved in 1926.[67] The Anglo-American model of training was so dominant within the ICN that the organization had no flexibility to adjust to the circumstances of various groups of nurses who were prepared for specialized tasks in a somewhat different way.

Karll's Philosophy and Vision

Karll advocated refocusing nurses' motherhouse traditions. In her eyes, nursing made ongoing contributions to the progress of humankind that were still rooted in the principles of service and religious faith. Nurses, she believed, had to broaden their perspective to give up the subservient and shortsighted morality so often learned in the motherhouses. This was one of Karll's most important motivations for translating Dock and Nutting's four-volume work, *A History of Nursing*, into German. The first volume of this history underscored the idea of progressive ethics. Karll abhorred any

physical exploitation or spiritual restriction on nurses. In her eyes, good nursing care required not only technical skills, but a developed personality and a broad mind that would be able to grasp the social needs of the time.[68] She believed that the most important role of future nurses would be to serve as "apostles of hygiene," promoters of social progress, not just to take care of the physical needs of patients.[69] In many ways Karll still spoke the language of devotion and service, as did the other influential nursing leaders of her time.[70]

Karll was concerned about nurses who idealistically undertook professional responsibility at very young ages, only to confront the harsh reality of the work, which quickly destroyed their personalities. After a few years, the nurses were "overworked, exhausted, [with] often disabled bodies and a broken spirit."[71] Though Karll believed nurses needed to retain the service motive, characterized by self-denial and self-sacrifice, she did not advocate the senseless destruction of nurses' physical and mental health. To establish social progress, nurses had to commit themselves and be responsible for improving their situation through the creation of a shared professional identity, which would encourage them to take responsibility for their own independence, protection, and professional opportunities.[72]

The Tragedy of German Nursing: World War I and Its Aftermath

During the First World War (1914–1918), Karll's leadership took on a new dimension. When the Red Cross refused the war service of the POGN, Karll contacted the Austrian war administration, which eagerly accepted Karll's help. With a large group of POGN nurses, she went to Austria and provided nursing service in the many hospitals and tuberculosis camps.

However, organized attempts to improve the condition of nursing stagnated with the First World War. Many German nurses were recruited for service or became unemployed during the war. After Germany's defeat, very high reparation payments devastated the economy, resulting in high inflation and high unemployment. Like its country, the POGN was financially devastated, with limited funds to maintain its organization. Without foreign support, the POGN would most certainly have folded. High unemployment among the nurses often resulted in hunger and homelessness. The French and Belgian occupation of the Ruhr area in 1923 worsened the situation as even more nurses lost their jobs.[73]

During the second half of the 1920s, the POGN was able to slowly reestablish itself. The journal, which had ceased publication until March 1924, began to reappear regularly. But Karll's own physical health was compromised after a mastectomy and radiation therapy in 1924; the 1925 ICN conference in Finland was the last ICN meeting she was able to attend. By 1926, Karll was considerably more debilitated and unable to continue her previous travel schedule. Essentially bedridden, she was cared for in one of the clinics in Berlin by her sister and many of her POGN nurses until she died in 1927. Shortly after her death, the POGN moved into the newly established Berlin office in 1928, which was called the "Agnes Karll House" in her honor.[74]

The movement toward an independent nursing organization, so energetically started by Karll and her colleagues, did not grow during the next decade; the POGN faced a grim political reality. The campaigns of the dawning Hitler era attracted many nurses to the "state union of German nurses" during the late 1920s. The membership of the POGN declined. The Nazi union idealized the feminine and motherly roles of the nurse, and through the motherhood cult of the Nazi propaganda, nurses were recruited to spread the ideology of the "health of the nation" with its eugenic, racist, and eventually murderous implications.[75] The POGN's journal was prohibited in 1933, and the organization itself was abolished in 1939.

After the Second World War, Helene Blunck, the last president before the war, reestablished the POGN as "Agnes Karll Verband" in the American and British allied areas. Eventually the Swedish ICN president, Gerda Hoyer, visiting Berlin in 1948, ensured Germany's reinvolvement with the ICN at the 1949 meeting in Stockholm.[76]

Conclusion

Karll's leadership reflected a strong commitment to the cause of independent nurses, the progress of humankind, and the creation of a new organization of nursing care. Having experienced the harsh reality of motherhouse apprenticeship and private duty nursing, she envisioned a way to improve the conditions of independent nurses. Her life-long interest in women's affairs and her support of the women's movement enabled her to bring her ideas of self-organization into effect for nurses. Although running a business was a new and unexplored area for women, Karll led the new nursing association with a keen and determined mind. She successfully

mobilized the interest of a private insurance company to financially support the new nursing organization and to provide a special insurance policy for nurses. Her energetic and charismatic leadership not only contributed to the successful establishment of the German nursing association and its nursing bureau, but helped to link German nursing with the worldwide community of nurses through the ICN. Tragically, Karll's plans for an independent nursing organization were cut short by her early death from breast cancer. The seeds of nursing independence and self-responsibility she had planted so carefully did not get a chance to flourish in the grim economic and political reality of Germany between the First and Second World Wars. Nevertheless, the development of the German nurses' association under her leadership mirrored the wider sociopolitical, economic, and cultural changes of early-twentieth-century Germany.

GEERTJE BOSCHMA
Doctoral Candidate
School of Nursing
University of Pennsylvania
Bottemaheerd 69
9737 NB Groningen
The Netherlands
Phone: 011 31 50 422823

Acknowledgments

I wish to thank Joan Lynaugh, Norma M. Lang, Barbara L. Brush, and Eileen Sullivan-Marx for their generous comments.

Notes

1. See "Records of Achievement—Sister Agnes Karll," *Trained Nurse and Hospital Review* 72, no. 2 (February 1924): 223 (hereafter cited as *TNHR*); and Agnes Karll, *Geschichte der fünf ersten Jahre unseres Verbandes* (Berlin: Deutscher Verlag, 1908), 1.

2. A. P. Kruse, *Die Krankenpflegeausbildung seit der Mitte des 19: Jahrhunderts* (Stuttgart: Kohlhammer, 1987), 69–105.

3. See Karll, 1; and Margarete Lungershausen, *Agnes Karll, Ihr Leben, Werk und Erbe* (Hannover: Elwin Staude Verlag, 1964), 13–17.

4. Lavinia L. Dock, "The Rise of the German Free Sisters," in *A History of Nursing,* ed. Adelaide Nutting and Lavinia L. Dock, vol. 4 (New York: G. P. Put-

nam's Sons, 1912), 7. Dock describes the efforts of independent nurses in Germany to establish themselves as a respected paid profession while breaking with the traditional restrictive congregational nursing system.

5. Karll, 1.

6. Hans Peter Schaper, *Krankenwartung und Krankenpflege. Tendenzen der Verberuflichung in der ersten Hälfte des 19 Jahrhunderts* (Opladen: Leske und Budrich, 1987), 75–79, 80–81.

7. Kruse, 38–39.

8. Irene Schuessler Poplin, *A Study of the Kaiserswerth Deaconess Institutes' Nurse Training School in 1850–1851: Purposes and Curriculum* (PhD diss., University of Texas at Austin, 1988), 40.

9. Dock, 4–5.

10. Poplin, 53–57, 276–317.

11. Kruse, 43–51.

12. See R. F. Nyrop, ed., *Federal Republic of Germany: a Country Study* (Washington, D.C.: U.S. Goverment, 1982) 16–19, for a discussion of Germany's industrial and population growth.

13. See Poplin, 25–29; and George Rosen, *A History of Public Health* (New York: M. C. Publications, 1958), 192ff.

14. During the nineteenth century, a liberal and later socialist movement developed in Germany. Within this context the women's movement fought for economic independence for women. This movement provided the framework for nurses to improve their situation, as the work of Agnes Karll demonstrates. See Lungershausen, 1–41.

15. It is a translation of the German phrase *"freien" oder "wilden" Schwestern* (free or wild nurses). Lungershausen, 13–14. Whereas in English "wild" would mean something like "not civilized" or "disturbed," in German this term means in this particular context only "not bound" or "established independently." The term is more neutral in German. Free nurses were not bound to any motherhouse; they worked independently for a salary. At the time it was controversial for middle- and upper-class women to do so. This group of free nurses grew in large cities in particular, and encompassed both untrained female ward attendants and women who had separated themselves from a motherhouse and now worked independently, usually as private duty nurses (Lungershausen, 13–14). This group was controversial because they worked for a living and lacked legal protection.

16. Dock, 7.

17. Ibid., 4–5.

18. Claudia Bischoff, *Frauen in der Krankenpflege: Zur Entwicklung von Frauenrolle und Frauenberufstätigkeit in 19 und 20 Jahrhundert* (Frankfurt am Main: Campus Verlag, 1984), 94–103, 108–109. Bischoff argues that the unprotected status of the independent nurses forced them to work long hours, often through the night with hardly any days off.

19. In German: Berufsorganisation der Krankenpflegerinnen Deutschlands. Usually abbreviated as BO. The organization is referred to as the POGN in this article, which is the abbreviation of the English translation.

20. For biographical information see Lavinia L. Dock, "An Appreciation —

Sister Agnes Karll," *American Journal of Nursing* 27, no. 5 (May 1927): 357–58; and Lungershausen, 19–20.

21. Lungershausen, 19. Karll describes the director of the school, Johanna Wilborn, as an advocate of women's emancipation and self-organization of teachers. Karll developed a longstanding friendship with her and owed to her the foundation of much of her later work.

22. See Lungershausen, 19–20; and Dock, "An Appreciation," 357–58.

23. Lungershausen, 19–20.

24. Karrl herself ascribed her breakdown to the hard labor conditions at the time. See Lungershausen, 19–20.

25. See Abraham Zaleznik, "What makes a leader?" *Success* (June 1989): 42–44, for a discussion of leadership qualities. Zaleznik argues that leadership qualities are developed as a result of conflicting experiences and an introspective capacity that reinforces creative problem solving.

26. Karll, 5–6.

27. Lungershausen, 39.

28. Karll, 6, 51.

29. Kruse, 16.

30. Nursing personnel were not included in state social security laws until 1923, and even then only partially. (Bischoff, 110.) Lungershausen, 15, argued that due to the motherhouse system in which nursing was viewed as an unselfish calling, nurses lacked the political influence to make their voices heard. Moreover, religious associations resisted state interference with their affairs. Changing the lack of protection for nurses was one of the goals of Karll's endeavor.

31. Karll, 6, 51.

32. Dock "An Appreciation," 358.

33. See Lungershausen, 15–16; and Dock, "An Appreciation," 357.

34. Karll, 5.

35. Lungershausen, 17.

36. An organized women's movement began in Germany during the revolutionary period of 1848. Democratic rights, education for women, and the social question remained central issues of women's organizations during the remainder of the nineteenth and beginning of the twentieth centuries. The League of German Womens' Associations (Bund Deutches Frauenvereine) was founded in 1894, advocating suffrage and access to higher education. Because of different views as to how to achieve these goals, a radical wing split off from the association in 1899. Within the GWA the political implications of a new feminist ethic were hotly debated. According to the new ethic, women in particular would be able to contribute to social progress because of their female characteristics. Civil rights and suffrage could increase women's role in public life and thus contribute to the betterment of society. Public hygiene and social reform were considered prime areas of women's work. Agnes Karll's view of nurses as promoters of social progress reflects this debate on feminist ethics within the German women's movement. For a discussion of the German women's movement, see Section IV of "Organisation und Politik," in *Frauen suchen ihre Geschichte*, ed. Karin Hausen (München: Beck, 1983), 196–275.

37. Karll, 5.

38. Lungershausen, 16.

39. Kruse, 52.

40. See Lungershausen, 13, 16; and Kruse, 51–54. Zimmer supported Agnes Karll and her friends in presenting their case to the Council of Women and agreed with them on the need for a state exam. He lobbied among government officials to establish a state examination for nurses. Furthermore, Zimmer founded the Schwesternschaft Deutscher Frauendienst (Sisterhood of German Women's Service), apparently a group of independent nursing schools. His daughter, Maria Zimmer, became superintendent of the largest of these (Lungershausen, 16).

41. Karll, 6. Karll noted that she would not have been able to afford these expenses herself.

42. Lungershausen, 17–18.

43. Karll, 6–7.

44. Lungershausen, 17–18.

45. Karll, 6.

46. The event clearly demonstrates how difficult it is to envision something new, to break with old forms if one is still grounded in them. Moreover, within the German women's movement there was just beginning to be an awareness of the importance of expanding female control over female professional and educational affairs. By the end of the nineteenth century, schools for girls, for example, were usually directed by men. See Irene Stoehr, "Organisierte Mütterlichkeit: Zur Politik der deutschen Frauenbewegung um 1900," in *Frauen suchen ihre Geschichte,* ed. Karin Hausen (München: Beck, 1983), 221–249, particularly 234.

47. Lungershausen, 23–26.

48. Karll, 49–50.

49. Karll, 10. In German: *denn von uns hatte noch nie jemand ein Protocoll aufgenommen, geschweige denn eine Versammlung geleitet.*

50. Lungershausen, 24–25.

51. Karll, *Geschichte ersten Jahre,* 12–16.

52. Dock, "The Rise," 26–27.

53. Karll, 11.

54. Karll, 66.

55. Dock, "An Appreciation," 358.

56. Lungershausen, 26.

57. As medicine became more successful and the number of hospitals expanded, the demand for nurses increased at the beginning of the century. Once the POGN had established its reputation, some hospitals began negotiating with the POGN to have their wards staffed with POGN nurses. In 1905, the first hospital directors of Düsseldorf approached Karll to negotiate POGN nurses' placement in one of their new hospitals. Other hospitals soon followed (Lungershausen, 36–37).

58. Agnes Karll to Lavinia Dock, 9 May 1907, Letters of Karll to Lavinia Dock, 1907–1912, Archives of the International Council of Nurses, Geneva, Switzerland (hereafter cited as ICN-Archives).

59. Lungershausen, 37–39.

60. Dock, "The Rise," 8–10.

61. Karll, *Geschichte ersten Jahre,* 24.

62. Karll to Lavinia Dock, 1907–1912, ICN-Archives.

63. Kruse, 69–103.

64. Lungershausen, 35.

65. Ibid., 36.

66. Ibid., 71–72.

67. Ibid., 72.

68. Ibid., 18–19. See also Karll, *Geschichte ersten Jahre*, 23.

69. Lungershausen, 30.

70. Diane Hamilton, "Constructing the Mind of Nursing," *Nursing History Review* 2 (1994): 3–28. Hamilton describes the core value of the nursing philosophy of Lavinia Dock, Lillian Wald, and Annie Goodrich as "compassion toward humanity" (p. 22). Hamilton further states that "they envisioned that secular nursing would emulate the values of religious sisters without accepting their rules, regulations, and cloistered life" (p. 22). Compassion would be based on a "commitment to the authority of humanity and its social progress" (p. 22).

71. Lungershausen, 9. In German: *einen überarbeiteten, erschöpften oft völlig siechen Körper und einen gebrochenen Geist.*

72. Karll, *Geschichte ersten Jahre*, 28, 44–46.

73. Agnes Karll, "Nursing in Germany During the Year 1923," International Council of Nurses' *Bulletin*, no. 1 (1924): 28–29.

74. Lungershausen, 55–56.

75. Hilde Steppe, *Krankenpflege im Nationalsozialismus* (Frankfurt am Main: Mabuse Verlag, 1989).

76. Lungershausen, 70–71.

DOING THE WORK OF HISTORY

The Diary as Historical Evidence
The Case of Sarah Gallop Gregg

KATHLEEN S. HANSON
College of Nursing
University of Illinois at Chicago

M. PATRICIA DONAHUE
College of Nursing
University of Iowa

Introduction

On 1 January 1863, Sarah Gallop Gregg, a milliner from Ottawa, Illinois, began two years of service as a nurse with the Union forces during the Civil War. During these years she recorded in her diary the events of the day. After the war, Sarah Gregg returned to Ottawa, where she remained until her death in 1897.[1] Knowledge of her Civil War service and of her diary lingered among local residents, but she was generally unknown outside of LaSalle County, Illinois. Her name briefly surfaced in 1929 and in the early 1930s, when she was represented in a collection of figurines by distinguished sculptress Mina Schmidt. The figurines, depicting women of note in Illinois history, were exhibited at the World's Columbian Exposition in 1929 and 1932.[2] Mrs. Gregg's name also appeared in two master's theses during the 1930s and in two articles in the *Journal of the Illinois State Historical Society*.[3] Mrs. Gregg again faded from public awareness. In 1968, Dr. R. C. Slater, an osteopath from LaSalle, Illinois, and a collector of Lincoln memorabilia, donated to the Illinois State Historical Library a typed manuscript of the Civil War diary of Sarah Gregg and photocopies of some of her

Nursing History Review 4 (1996): 169–86. Copyright © 1996 by The American Association for the History of Nursing.

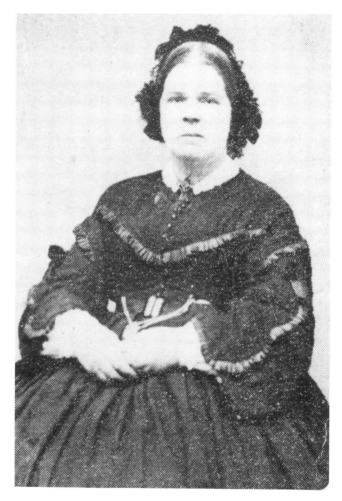

Figure 1. Sarah Gallop Gregg. (Courtesy of the Illinois State Historical Library)

correspondence.[4] These materials were unused until a group of school-children began a local history project.

In 1985, four eighth-grade students from the Springfield, Illinois, area conducted a local history project on Camp Butler, a nearby Civil War train-ing camp, and discovered the manuscript of the diary of Sarah Gregg, a Civil War nurse, among state archival materials.[5] The town newspaper reported this find, and the article was forwarded to the first author (KH). By such serendipitous ways came the raw material for historical research.

The location of material is only the beginning step for the historian. The finding of new primary source data is not valuable in and of itself; it requires the rigorous and systematic approach of historical methodology to yield that which is called history. A diary, and in this particular case the manuscript of a diary, presents some unique challenges to researchers.

Purposes

This article has three major purposes: (1) to discuss the credibility of diaries as primary evidence for historical research, (2) to discuss the usefulness of diaries to historians, and (3) to illustrate the methodology of verification using the diary of Sarah Gregg, Civil War nurse.

The writing of diaries is an old practice that can be traced as far back as the sixteenth century. Diaries have been an important part of the American culture since a wave of colonists migrated to New England in the 1630s.[6] As sources of historical evidence, diaries can be extremely useful in a variety of ways. They can provide examples of contemporary opinion, vivid details that allow for the visualization of historical situations, knowledge acquisition and value shifts that occur in life, and firsthand evidence for happenings of questionable historicity. In essence, diaries can link the reader of today with the writer of the past "with intimate threads and exhibit as nothing else can the unbroken consecutive flow of human endeavor, failure, and hope."[7] Although the use of diaries in contemporary works is once again gaining in popularity and recognition as more than pure reproductions of the originals, few publications are available that analyze the various criteria and processes that must be employed in the appraisal of their credibility.[8]

Credibility of Diaries as Primary Evidence for Historical Research

Diaries are one form of historical evidence regarded as primary or original works, those sources that existed at the time the historical event was happening and that aid in its description. Frequently, however, there is an underlying assumption that everyone knows and agrees on what a diary is. Yet there is difficulty in finding a definition that clearly distinguishes diaries from other forms of writing such as journals, autobiographies, and memoirs.

Definitions of diaries, which often depend on the intended use of the diaries, can be both narrow or expansive, ranging from the simple "record of events or thoughts written as dated periodic entries"[9] to the more complex "personal record of what interested the diarist, usually kept day by day, each day's record being self-contained and written soon after the events occurred, the style usually being free from organized exposition."[10] The stable factor in all definitions is that entries of personal thoughts and experiences are assumed to be recorded on the same day that they occurred. Journals, on the other hand, are usually defined as those official records related to jobs or personal recordings that focus on internal rather than external concerns.[11] In a number of instances, journals are referred to as the more intimate writing; in other cases, authors refer to diaries as the more intimate. Thus, the question of a distinction between diaries and journals may be moot and entirely dependent on their purpose. One might even go so far as to say that the terms are hopelessly muddled.

Memoirs and autobiographies are also regarded as primary sources and are frequently discussed in relation to diaries and journals. They are based to a great extent on memory and are usually considered to be of the same class or category of historical account. According to G. J. Garraghan, there is merely an "accidental difference" between the two; an autobiography usually embraces the individual's entire life or career, while a memoir may cover only a part of the participation in an event or series of events.[12] Diaries are distinguished from memoirs by the fact that they are kept more or less as events occur rather than composed long after the events have happened. Thus, diaries are considered to be eyewitness accounts of personal experiences and external phenomena written under the immediate influence of experience, and, as such, are more reliable.[13]

Garraghan distinguishes two types of diaries: the intimate or introspective, and the factual or objective.[14] The intimate diary reveals inner thoughts and feelings of the writer and may also contain daydreams, fantasies, and moral inclinations. The factual diary primarily records external happenings, although personal thoughts and feelings may be obliquely evident. Diaries may also be classified according to regional practices such as that described in *A Midwife's Tale*. Ulrich explains that in eighteenth-century New England, daybooks and the interleaved almanac were used for record keeping. The former were economic entries that were sometimes combined with notes on significant family events; the latter was a record of a variety of things such as the weather, visits to and from neighbors, and public events. It is also feasible that an individual's diary might be a com-

bination of types, as was the case with the diary of Martha Ballard, the midwife.[15] Furthermore, the elements of value in a diary are oftentimes dependent on the particular discipline. For psychologists, a personal document (diary/journal) is a self-revealing record of the author's mental life, which is extremely useful when spontaneous and intimate.[16] The social historian, on the other hand, values the diary for its objective and subjective contributions. Firsthand descriptions and illustrations of the conditions and customs of the time constitute objective contributions. The subjective descriptions reveal the philosophy, ideals, and the soul of the writer.[17]

It is clear that there are numerous types, classifications, and uses of diaries. They are used by scholars, teachers, and students in disciplines such as anthropology, sociology, psychology, literature, political science, and history. The importance or value of diaries to these individuals may vary, and their purpose may be similar or quite different. The fact remains, however, that the use of diaries as an art form and contributor to an understanding of humanity and particular phases of social life and events remains relatively untapped.

Diaries and Historians

As early as 1921, diaries were considered to be among the most important documents used by historians.[18] They derived their chief merit as historical source from the fact that they are records, often in vivid detail, made at the same time that personal experiences and events happen. In other words, their spontaneity and intimacy contribute to their value.[19] In this regard, they can reveal human nature in a way that is unattainable in any other form of writing: they depict the pleasures and miseries of everyday life, render illustrations of manners and customs that have disappeared, provide archeological information about places or people, and disclose examples of contemporary opinion.[20]

Diaries furnish historians with facts about people, places, and events (public, private, political, and social). Barzun and Graff, in their discussion of evidences of historical truth, consider diaries to be intentional transmitters of facts. In other words, diary authors specifically intend their words to record a part of history for future use.[21] Facts from diaries can supply vivid detail that enables historians to visualize historical situations and determine their position in the context of the times. In many cases, they provide conclusive, firsthand evidence of happenings of questionable historicity or

of circumstances in which data have been left partially obscured.[22] In addition, diary entries may be useful in establishing unknown or doubtful dates.

Of particular significance is the worth of diaries in preserving information about events and individuals of the past. This aspect of preservation is extremely important to historians whose primary data are generally preserved documents or artifacts. But beyond the documents and diaries themselves, preservation also involves other elements that may be equally or more important. These include "the gradual acquisition of knowledge and shifting of values that occur in life."[23] This is consistent with the belief by a school of historians who "contend that values and ideas change with periods of history, that what is a justifiable principle of esthetics, morality, and politics at one time may be less so at another, that thought patterns are relative to contemporary conditions arising out of the cultural and historical climate of a given area and time. That belief, which would deny the validity of absolute principles in history, is sometimes called *historical relationism* or *historicism*."[24] The value of diaries to historians or other scholars can usually be placed in one of the two categories, objective contributions or subjective contributions, which have been previously described. According to Van der Velde, it is the latter category that is especially valuable in situations where the diary writer may be considered an influential leader or typical of a large group.[25]

WOMEN'S LIVES AND WOMEN'S WORK
Attention is now being given to the large gaps in women's histories, which have been sparse prior to the twentieth century. According to contemporary thought, an analysis of women's life writings, including diaries, can fill these gaps and transform society's understanding of history by providing a view of history through the eyes of women and ordered by values they define, rendering accounts of history based on the experiences of women, contributing a view of history potentially different from that of a male-oriented society, and reinterpreting the past in light of women's cultural milieu.[26] In other words, "A study of diaries may reformulate our ideas of how ordinary women spoke, thought and perceived their worlds."[27]

Although women have had a long history of diary writing, their diaries were frequently dismissed as being trivial and unimportant. Descriptions of domestic chores, pastimes, family responsibilities, the weather, and inner feelings were considered mundane or ordinary and thus incapable of contributing to an understanding of American history. These diaries were taken seriously only when either the times or individuals were considered to be extraordinary.

Typically, the writings of women have been read primarily by women and were either ridiculed or ignored by White male historians or considered to be outside the interest of most scholars. Only in certain circumstances, such as the suffrage movement and other prominently female reform movements, have the contributions and achievements of women been noted and incorporated within historical texts. Yet women have chronicled many events of great national importance in their diaries. For example, the most distinct and significant group of American diaries written in the last half of the nineteenth century dealt with the Civil War.[28]

Contemporary feminism has facilitated the rising importance of women's diaries, which have become prominent for historical and literary purposes, as well as for use in women's studies. This increasing interest in the lives, contributions, and achievements of women has also led to the development of several outstanding female historians and the growing availability of source materials.[29] Through these efforts, history "as a dynamic process of reinterpreting the past in light of the contemporary cultural milieu and the availability of new evidence" may be demonstrated.[30]

PROBLEMS WITH DIARIES

Problems with the use of diaries for historical research can be created by the diarist, the diary editor, the publisher, family members, or the historian. At times, a combination of these may exist according to the circumstances surrounding a particular diary. The fact remains that all diarists are selective. The distinctly personal character of a diary leads to the probability of subjectivism or bias that may be at cross-purposes with the actual truth.[31] In addition, diaries may be kept for a specific purpose — for public consumption or for the justification of self. In the latter case, spontaneity may be greatly reduced.[32] Finally, there are instances in which gaps are filled in by the diarist at a later time. These particular entries, then, were not made on the assigned dates but are based on recollections or on other sources.[33]

The preservation and publication of diaries may also raise problems. An editor may be overly zealous to protect the diarist and family members, and seek to eliminate all potentially discrediting material. Distortion of the text may thus occur, since the published diary may be reconstructed and the modifications hidden until the historian examines the original manuscript, usually at a later time. This may be particularly true in totalitarian countries when diaries incorporate information about contemporary political crises and events, and names of individuals may have to be disguised to avoid retaliation.[34]

Diaries as primary source material can present a challenge to histo-

rians. In addition to the difficulties previously described, the historian may also be faced with the problem of accessibility. Once accessibility has been achieved, however, other difficulties present themselves by virtue of the fact that most historians must deal with diaries of individuals who are dead and cannot be cross-examined about the diary's specific content. The historian is unable to substantiate through personal contact the authenticity of the diary, the competence of the diarist, the completeness of the diary, or the meaning of the contents. Gottschalk's discussion of the use of personal documents clearly demonstrates these difficulties — since the diarist cannot be asked whether parts of the diary are based on personal experience or whether the diarist is absolutely positive about information that contradicts other evidence. Information cannot be clarified, missing elements in the narrative cannot be provided, and the specific motive for writing cannot be ascertained.[35] Therefore, it is critical that the historian be extremely careful in the analysis of the diary, since the danger of inaccurate interpretation or overinterpretation does exist.[36]

It is also imperative that the historian maintain the rigor of historical method when dealing with a diary, just as with any other type of personal document. Examining, testing, and using the documents are the crux of the issue. In other words, the central questions for historical research data are "questions of verification, of analysis, and then of synthesis."[37]

Verification of the Diary

Since Sarah Gregg's original diary was not a part of the archival material, could the accuracy of the content of the manuscript be determined? Barzun and Graff suggest that every thinking person must learn to discriminate between "what is true and what is false, what is probable and what is doubtful or impossible."[38] The historian, however, must reach a conclusion that is convincing to him- or herself and to others. The method by which this is done is called *verification*. According to Barzun and Graff, verification involves a combination of researcher skills and attributes and a series of processes or techniques by which useful historical information is drawn from the raw material. The qualities the historian brings to the process are the ability to note details, common-sense reasoning, a developed "feel" for history, a familiarity with human behavior, and ever-enlarging stores of information. The techniques and processes include (1) *collation* — matching copies with sources; (2) dealing with *rumor, legend,* and *fraud;* (3) *attribu-*

tion — putting a name to a source; (4) *explication* — decoding and classifying documents; and (5) *disentanglement, clarification,* and *identification* — ascertaining worth through authorship.[39] These processes are not applied in a lock-step manner, but are fluid, allowing the researcher to move back and forth in the raw material and to work on various levels of analyses. Verification, or determining that which is true and probable, became the central focus of the researchers' initial work on Sarah Gregg, Civil War nurse.

The application of the processes of collation and attribution to the Sarah Gregg diary illustrates the movement between levels of analysis as the historian works with the raw material. Collation is the technique of matching copies with sources; attribution is the technique of putting a name to a source. In the case of the Sarah Gregg diary, collation occurred on two levels. The first level, and the least complex, involved matching the typed manuscript in the Illinois State Historical Library archives with the researchers' copy of the manuscript.[40] The second level of collation, matching the entries of the typed manuscript with diary entries found in other documents, was more critical to the researchers' use of the diary as historical material.

The Illinois State Historical Library is in possession of the typed manuscript noted as the diary entries of Sarah Gregg. The current location of the *original* diary is unknown. The authenticity and accuracy of the typed manuscript is thus questionable unless a comparison with the original is made. Three approaches to this second level of collation were formulated: (1) a genealogical search to locate descendants of Sarah Gregg who might have knowledge of the location of the original diary, (2) a search for information on A. Tisler (the name of the person on the typed manuscript, presumed to be the person who typed the manuscript), and (3) a search for information on the original diary of Sarah Gregg in her hometown of Ottawa, Illinois.

To date, the genealogical search has been unsuccessful. The location of the original diary remains unknown. Efforts to find more information regarding the typed manuscript have been more fruitful. The Tisler family, along with the Greggs, were residents of Ottawa, Illinois, from 1850 through the early 1900s. No connection by marriage between the families was found, but it is obvious that they and their descendants were acquainted. Charles B. Tisler and Catherine Tisler emigrated to the United States from France, arriving in New York and settling in Ottawa, Illinois, in 1855. Catherine Tisler died in 1867, and Charles B. Tisler died in 1895. Their son, Frederick, began his working career as a carpenter and was

employed in the construction of many buildings in Ottawa. Among his children was a daughter, Adel L. Tisler, perhaps the A. Tisler who transcribed the Sarah Gregg diary.[41] David R. and Sarah Gregg moved to Ottawa, Illinois, in 1848. David Gregg was a carpenter and joiner, and Sarah owned a millinery shop. Their son, William P. Gregg, was a paperhanger. Both Frederick Tisler and William Gregg were members of the Ancient Order of United Workers.[42] Another connection between the Tisler family and the Sarah Gregg diary is evidenced by an inclusion of diary excerpts in a publication by Charles C. Tisler in 1939. Included in this small collection of poems and prose is a selection entitled "Mrs. Gregg's Diary Tells of Wartime Fourth," describing her service as Civil War nurse and matron of the Camp Butler hospital, and the quotation of seven diary entries.[43] The quotations in the 1939 publication, which may or may not have preceded the typed manuscript, corresponded exactly with the diary entries for the same dates in the typed manuscript. It was concluded that there was correspondence in the accuracy of diary entries among the materials associated with the Tislers and that it was very probable that the Tislers had access to the original diary.

The third approach was to locate other material regarding the diary from sources in the Ottawa, Illinois, area. Again this approach was fruitful. The LaSalle County Historical Society proved to be a source of information for the researchers. Information on Sarah Gregg or the Gregg family was not directly indexed in their materials; however, materials on the early years of the town of Ottawa contained material on the Greggs and the diary. Among these materials was a 1912 publication by the local newspaper entitled *Ottawa: Old and New*. This small book was a compilation of newspaper articles and clippings that chronicled the development of the town and the lives of many of the citizens. There were several entries on the Gregg family members; however, one entry on Sarah Gregg and her Civil War activities was particularly useful in the process of matching diary copies.[44] The article referred to the diary that Mrs. Gregg kept during her service as a nurse in the Civil War and directly quoted six entries, two undated entries and four dated. The entries in the newspaper article corresponded directly with the entries in the typed manuscript.[45] A total of thirteen different diary entries were located in other documents; all thirteen corresponded with the typed manuscript.

The process of matching copies yielded information the researchers were able to use in the verification processes of attribution (putting a name to a source) and identification (ascertaining worth through authorship).

As Barzun and Graff note, the probability of truth is often built by the cumulation of evidence, with each item reinforcing the genuineness of the next. In situations in which direct evidence is unavailable, a concurrence of indirect evidence can establish truth.[46] The biographical sketches of the Tisler and Gregg families; the confirmation of the existence of Sarah Gregg's diary in both the Tisler publication and the *Republican-Times* newspaper articles; and the correspondence of the quotations of the diary entries in the Tisler publication, the *Republican-Times* articles, and the typed manuscript in the state historical collection led the researchers to conclude that the typed manuscript is an accurate, if not complete, transcription of the diary of Sarah Gregg.

Diaries are by their very nature replete with many incidents that encourage the researcher to question whether an event really occurred or whether the event occurred as the diarist portrayed. Barzun and Graff suggest that it is as difficult to judge when to be skeptical about the small events as it is to question the "too pat" legend. The researcher's own fund of knowledge about an era, particularly an understanding of people's behavior, beliefs, and lifestyles, provides the background against which the raw material is juxtaposed. The more knowledge the researcher possesses, the more questions are raised. There were many incidents in the Sarah Gregg diary that caused the researchers to wonder whether the event occurred or if it occurred as reported. The role Sarah Gregg played as a nurse aboard the steamer "City of Alton" was such an example. It seemed almost too providential that her experiences as a nurse encompassed every possible role: visitor at the hospitals at Cairo, nurse at a local training camp, matron at Camp Butler, and service aboard a hospital transport. Yet she remained unknown in nursing and Civil War history. A variety of sources had corroborated the experiences as visitor, training camp nurse, and hospital matron.[47] The diary, however, was the only source for her involvement on the hospital transport "City of Alton." Again the process of verification called for multiple approaches: (1) substantiating the use of the "City of Alton" as a hospital transport ship on the Mississippi at the time of the siege of Vicksburg, (2) determining the accuracy of Mrs. Gregg's account of the trip, and (3) corroborating the presence of Mrs. Gregg on the steamer.

The official records of the Civil War and general histories of the war do not list the "City of Alton" as a part of the army hospital transport system on the Mississippi. The lack of inclusion in the official records was not particularly alarming, since the management of the sick and wounded soldiers did not lie solely with the army and federal government agencies. Individ-

ual state governors had the authority to charter and commission local ships for service with state militia. According to the Gregg diary, Governor Yates chartered the "City of Alton" to travel from Cairo to Vicksburg to pick up wounded.[48] No records of the "City of Alton" as a hospital ship were found in the state historical library; however, an undated photograph of the ship was located. The Sarah Gregg diary indicates that the steamer unloaded its wounded at St. Louis. Documents on file at the Missouri State Historical Society verify the use of the "City of Alton" as a transport steamer carrying Grant's Army of the Tennessee south, the ship's presence at the Battle of Shiloh, and the removal of wounded from Pittsburgh Landing to hospitals in St. Louis during April of 1862.[49] These documents indicated the steamer was then returned to civilian shipping service. This army service preceded the Gregg diary entries by a year.

The reference to the hospitals in St. Louis prompted the researchers' recollection of the accounts of other nurses who served on hospital transport ships on the Mississippi. Emily E. Parsons was a Massachusetts woman who served as a Sanitary Commission nurse in St. Louis. Among her experiences described in L. P. Brockett's book on the role of women in the Civil War was a reference to being placed as head nurse on the hospital steamer "City of Alton." Miss Parson's trip on the steamer in January of 1863 was to pick up sick and wounded from Vicksburg and take them to hospitals at Memphis and St. Louis. These accounts gave ample evidence that the "City of Alton" had been used for hospital transport and that such usage spanned the time between the Battle of Shiloh in the spring of 1862 and the siege of Vicksburg in 1863. Although no definitive documentation of the trip in June 1863, as noted in the Gregg diary, has been found in official documents, a letter published in the *Ottawa Republican* on 13 June 1863 describes the trip of an Ottawa surgeon aboard the steamer "City of Alton" to pick up wounded at Vicksburg. This letter corresponds with Sarah Gregg's diary entry of 1 June 1863.[50] This letter was further used to verify the accuracy of Mrs. Gregg's account of the trip and the sequence of landings. Mrs. Gregg's account is more detailed, giving specific descriptions of sightings along the river and people encountered. The descriptions are an accurate representation of the geography of the river, and the encounters of various army personnel correspond to the placement of troops as recorded in the *Official Records of the War*.[51] No other sources identifying the presence of Mrs. Gregg aboard the steamer have been located. The researchers have concluded by these processes that the "City of Alton" was used as a hospital transport ship on the Mississippi during the Vicksburg campaign and that a surgeon from Ottawa was present on the ship during the June 1863 trip to

Vicksburg. The details given in the Gregg diary are probably an accurate account of that trip and support the diary claim that Sarah Gregg was recruited for such a trip, along with the local surgeon.

Conclusion

Diaries are credible sources of primary data for historians; however, their use must be tempered by an understanding of the purpose for which they were written. Diaries provide historical researchers with examples of contemporary opinion, vivid details that allow for the visualization of historical events, evidence of shifts in knowledge and values, and firsthand evidence of events of questionable historicity. Diaries are particularly useful in articulating the woman's perspective of events, which is so frequently missing from general history. Diaries, however, present the researcher with unique methodological problems.

The process of verification is a tool the historian uses to deal with the problems presented by a diary or its copy. The Sarah Gregg diary provided an opportunity to illustrate the use of these processes and establish the historical worth of the document. The cumulation of evidence suggested that the manuscript of the diary located in the archives of the Illinois State Historical Society is probably an accurate, but not necessarily complete, transcription of the original diary. As such, further study of the diary may shed more light on a woman's view of the American Civil War and the daily living activities of Civil War nurses.

KATHLEEN S. HANSON, PhD, RN
Assistant Professor
College of Nursing
University of Illinois at Chicago
Quad-Cities Regional Program
Suite 202
2525 Twenty-fourth Street
Rock Island, Illinois 61202
Phone: (309) 788-0844

M. PATRICIA DONAHUE, PhD, RN
Professor
College of Nursing
University of Iowa
Iowa City, Iowa 52242
Phone: (319) 354-7150

Acknowledgments

The research for this paper was supported by a Biomedical Research Support Grant, #2 So7 RR05776-10, Division of Research Resources, National Institutes of Health.

Notes

1. "Mrs. Sarah Gregg Dead," *Republican-Times,* 27 May 1897. The obituary of Sarah Gregg contained information on her early life but also included references to her contributions to the Civil War effort as a nurse and to the diary she kept.
2. "Mrs. Sarah Gregg," in *Brief Biographies of the Figurines on Display in the Illinois State Historical Library,* ed. Georgia L. Osborne and Emma B. Scott (Springfield: State of Illinois, 1932), 72. The figurines are a part of the Illinois State Historical collection because they represent the work of the artisan, Mina Schmidt, not because they represent historical women of Illinois. Other women who contributed to the Civil War effort were included in the collection and in the accompanying biographical sketches.
3. See Esther Vivian Hill, "Illinois Women in Soldier Welfare," (unpublished master's thesis, University of Illinois, 1934); Emma Eliza Parrote, "History of Camp Butler," (unpublished master's thesis, Butler University, 1938); William I. Kincaid, "Camp Butler," *Journal of the Illinois State Historical Society* 14 (April–July 1921): 382–85; and Helen Edith Sheppley, "Camp Butler in the Civil War Days," *Journal of the Illinois State Historical Society* 25 (n.d.): 285–317.
4. This material was gleaned from the card file entry for the Sarah Gregg diary at the Illinois Historical Library in Springfield, Illinois.
5. D. Pokorski, "Kids Dive into Archives and Come Out Winners," *State Journal Register,* 3 June 1985.
6. See H. Blodgett, *Centuries of Female Days: Englishwomen's Private Diaries,* (New Jersey: Rutgers University Press, 1988); S. E. Kagle, *American Diary Literature 1620–1799* (Boston: Twayne Publishers, 1979); S. E. Kagle, *Early Nineteenth-Century American Diary* (Boston: Twayne Publishers, 1986); W. Mathews, *American Diaries: An Annotated Bibliography of American Diaries Written Prior to the Year 1861* (Berkeley and Los Angeles: University of California Press, 1945); W. Mathews, *American Diaries in Manuscript 1580–1954, A Descriptive Bibliography,* (Athens: University of Georgia Press, 1974); K. O'Brien, *English Diaries and Journals* (London: William Collins of London, 1943); and A. Ponsonby, *English Diaries. A Review of English Diaries from the Sixteenth to the Twentieth Century with an Introduction of Diary Writing* (London: Methuen & Co., 1923). Motives for the writing of diaries are varied. Diaries are often created due to some disequilibrium in the author's life such as a spiritual crisis, some type of conflict, a journey, or significant events like wars. Kagle, for example, developed categories for diaries based on their types and uses: spiritual, travel/exploration, romance and courtship, war, and life/situation. Prior to the Civil War in America, a number of distinguished writers kept diaries, includ-

ing Alcott, Brown, Bryant, Cooper, Emerson, Longfellow, Melville, Thoreau, and Whitman.

7. Ponsonby, 43.

8. See M. M. Culpepper, *Trials and Triumphs, Women of the American Civil War* (East Lansing: Michigan State University Press, 1991); M. C. Gwin, *A Woman's Civil War* (Madison: University of Wisconsin Press, 1992; L. T. Ulrich, *A Midwife's Tale, The Life of Martha Ballard Based on Her Diary, 1785–1812* (New York: Alfred A. Knopf, 1990); and C. Vann Woodward, *Mary Chesnut's Civil War* (New Haven: Yale University Press, 1981).

9. Kagle, *American Diary Literature*, 15.

10. W. Mathews, *British Diaries: An Annotated Bibliography of British Diaries Written Between 1442 and 1942* (Berkeley and Los Angeles: University of California Press, 1950), xv.

11. The terms *journal* and *diary* are frequently used interchangeably and thus may cause some confusion to readers. This is perhaps due to the fact that there is a very fine distinction, if any, between the two. Although some authors may attempt to explain this distinction, they frequently resort to using them synonymously. See, for example, Blodgett, 1–62; G. J. Garraghan, *A Guide to Historical Method* (New York: Fordham University Press, 1988), 248–51; L. Gottschalk, *Understanding History, A Primer of Historical Method* (New York: Alfred A. Knopf, 1969), 94–95; Gwin, 3–18; Kagle, *American Diary Literature*, 15–24; and Ponsonby, 5.

12. Garraghan, 244–49. Frequently an author will use personal letters, diaries, and journals to aid with recall about experiences when preparing memoirs or autobiographies.

13. Allport specifies advantages of the diary as opposed to an autobiography. He contends that the diary can be particularly effective in capturing mood changes. In addition, diaries escape errors of memory as well as inappropriate interpretations of thoughts and feelings to which autobiographies and memoirs are prone. See G. W. Allport, *The Use of Personal Documents in Psychological Science* (New York: Social Science Research Council, 1941), 95–98.

14. Garraghan, 248–49.

15. Ulrich, 8.

16. Allport, 95.

17. L. G. Van der Velde, "The Diary of George Daffield," *Mississippi Valley Historical Review* 24 (n.d.): 25.

18. A. F. Pollard, "An Essay in Historical Method: The Barbellion Diaries," *History* (April 1921): 23. This author, however, cautions that this importance of the diary as raw material for the historian must be balanced with a method for testing and establishing genuineness and veracity in the document.

19. See Garraghan, 248–49; Gottschalk, 94–95; and L. Gottschalk, C. Kluckhohn, and R. Angell, *The Use of Personal Documents in History, Anthropology, and Sociology* (New York: Social Science Research Council, 1945), 18–19.

20. Ponsonby specifies that one way of estimating the value of a diary is by the light it throws on recorded incidents. He states that through an examination of such incidents in old diaries, "footnotes, amplifications and even new material for history have been discovered." See Ponsonby, 30; and Van der Velde.

21. J. Barzun and H. F. Graff, *The Modern Researcher* (New York: Harcourt, Brace & World, 1957), 132–33.

22. Garraghan, 248–50.

23. Kagle, *American Diary Literature,* 15. See also Kagle, *Early Nineteenth-Century.* This author renders perhaps the most comprehensive discussion of the evolution of diaries in America. His discussion includes valuable information on the motives for diary writing, the types and uses of diaries, and their significance in the understanding of shifting values and customs in America as well as emphasis on the changes in diary form related to "almost all of the major political, social, and artistic movements."

24. Gottschalk, Kluckhohn, and Angell, 25.

25. See Van der Velde.

26. For a more detailed discussion of the use of women's diaries as a means of presenting and explicating history as women's cultural experience, see the following: Blodgett; D. V. Gawronski, *History, Meaning and Method,* 3rd ed. (Glenview, Ill.: Scott, Foresman and Company, 1975); Gwin, 8–18; J. N. Lensink, "Expanding the Boundaries of Criticism: The Diary as Female Autobiography," *Women's Studies* 14:39; and Ulrich, 25–35.

27. Lensink, 44. Lensink strongly emphasizes the importance of female diaries. She argues that as more is learned about female psychology, language, and historical experience by such theorists as Carol Gilligan and Carroll Smith-Rosenburg, the diary will emerge as a female text. She believes that through diary writing, women have made their experiential lives coherent.

28. Kagle, *Early Nineteenth-Century,* 146. According to the author, the most distinguished group of diaries was written by Southern women. Other Civil War diaries were written by men (some soldiers).

29. Prominent female historians include Gerda Lerner, Ann Firor Scott, Julia Cherry Spruill, Mary Beard, Susan Reverby, and Barbara Melosh.

30. Gawronski, 94.

31. Numerous writers comment on these aspects of selectivity and subjectivism. See, for example, Blodgett; M. Culley, *A Day at a Time: The Diary Literature of American Women from 1764 to the Present* (New York: The Feminist Press, 1985); Garrigan; Gottschalk; and Ponsonby. Culley believes that all diarists are involved in a process in which they select details to create a "persona." She admits, however, that this process may be substantially unconscious. Ponsonby explains that the diarist must go through a process of "sifting and selection." Since it is impossible to record everything, the diarist chooses incidents which he or she believes matter at the particular moment in time. Thus, selectivity could be viewed as both an asset and a disadvantage.

32. C. Vann Woodward, in the introduction to *Mary Chesnut's Civil War,* carefully describes the alteration of the tone and the frankness with which Mary discusses events and people in her original journals as compared to the manuscript later published as her diary. The original journals, according to Vann Woodward, were clearly intended for Mary's private use and not open to scrutiny by even her husband. In her published book she states that her journal was frequently read by others. If that were the actual case, it could be construed that Mary Chesnut allowed

the journal to be read and that there was purpose behind the content of the entries. See C. Vann Woodward.

33. Gottschalk states that diaries or journals that contain such entries should more accurately be designated as memoirs. See Gottschalk, 95.

34. Gottschalk, 95.

35. Gottschalk, Kluckhorn, and Angell, 19–21.

36. Kagle, *American Diary Literature*, 18.

37. Gottschalk, Kluckhohn, and Angell, p. x.

38. J. Barzun and H. F. Graff, *The Modern Researcher*, 3rd ed. (San Diego: Harcourt Brace Jovanovich, 1977), 83.

39. Barzun and Graff, 3rd ed., 83–110.

40. In most instances, the modern historian uses the technology of photocopying to acquire accurate copies of primary data in the possession of others. Since the Illinois State Historical Library did not have the original diary of Sarah Gregg, nor was its location known, the accuracy of the typed manuscript could not be verified, so the library would not allow the researchers to photocopy it. The researchers, therefore, made audio recordings of the manuscript which were later transcribed. The researchers' transcript was then compared to the manuscript in the archives for accuracy in text, spelling, and punctuation.

41. *Biographical and Genealogical Records of LaSalle and Grundy Counties, Illinois* (Chicago: Lewis Publishing, 1900).

42. *History of LaSalle County, Illinois,* vol. I (Chicago: Inter-State Publishing, 1886).

43. C. C. Tisler, *Ramblin Around* (Ottawa, Ill.: Illinois Office Supply Company, 1939), 32–33.

44. *Ottawa: Old and New,* (Ottawa, Ill.: Republican Times, 1912–1914), 113–14.

45. The diary dates quoted in the newspaper article are as follows: 21 February 1865, 22 February 1865, 14 April 1865, and 16 April 1865. One of the undated entries corresponds to the last sentence of the 16 January 1863 entry in the typed manuscript; the second corresponds to a summary of an undated portion of the diary between 20 June 1863 and 26 December 1863.

46. Barzun and Graff, 3rd ed., 92–93.

47. See Kincaid, Shepply, Hill, and Parrote. Further data on Sarah Gregg's Civil War service are located in her pension file at the National Archives. See Sarah Gallop Gregg, Pension File, CAN no. 6912, bundle no. 25, National Archives.

48. The steamer "City of Alton" was used for a variety of purposes during the western campaign of the Civil War. Although the official records indicate the steamer was used to transport troops, horses, and supplies downriver during the siege of Vicksburg, the records are vague about the uses of the boat on trips upstream. Correspondence between Confederate officials Captain J. K. P. Pritchard, Acting Quartermaster, and Major L. A. Maclean, Assistant Adjutant General, include reference to the "City of Alton" traveling upriver from Vicksburg with a light load among boats that were either hospitals or empty. See J. K. P. Pritchard, "Captain to Major L. A. Maclean, 18 June 1863," in *The War of the Rebellion: A Compilation of the Official Records of the Union and Confederate Armies,* series I, vol. 22 (Wash-

ington, D.C.: GPO, 1901), 876–77. It is interesting to note that the "City of Alton" was used as a hospital transport in the spring 1864 Virginia Campaign. She sailed from Port Royal, Virginia, on 27 May 1864 with 700 wounded for hospitals in Washington, D.C. See *The War of the Rebellion* series I, vol. 36, 238–41.

49. References to the "City of Alton" at the Battle of Shiloh were found among the files of Missouri Historical Society. These files do not indicate all the original sources, but are part of a card index under the title "steamboats." Reference to the use of hospital transport ships on the Mississippi is found in Mrs. A. H. Hoge, *The Boys in Blue; Heroes of the "Rank and File"* (New York: E. B. Treat & Co., 1867), 64–71.

50. "Letter from a Surgeon," *Ottawa Republican Times*, 13 June 1863, substantiates Sarah Gregg's diary entry on 1 June 1863: "today Judge Cavalry called on us to procure a surgeon and two nurses to start within two hours to Cairo and meet the steamer which had been chartered and hospital boat to go down to Vicksburg and collect and bring all sick and wounded of the Union that could be found and bring them to northern hospitals. Accordingly in two hours from notice being given myself and husband reported at the Rock Island depot and started for Cairo."

51. Sarah Gregg's identification of islands in the river and the location of riverside towns was compared to maps of the Mississippi during the years 1860–1865. See *Echoes of Glory, Illustrated Atlas of the Civil War* (Alexandria, Va.: Time-Life Books, 1991), 217–29. The placement of troops as described in the Gregg diary was compared to histories of the siege of Vicksburg and to the official records of the war. See *The War of the Rebellion*, series I, vol. 22; and *Echoes of Glory, Illustrated Atlas*, 220–29.

BOOK REVIEWS

Suggestions for Thought by Florence Nightingale: Selections and Commentaries
Edited by Michael D. Calabria and Janet A. Macrae
(Philadelphia: University of Pennsylvania Press, 1994)

This book is an excellent resource for readers seeking to understand Florence Nightingale's thought and its place in the intellectual and philosophical history of nursing. The editors state in the preface that the volume is designed "to make the essence of Nightingale's spiritual philosophy accessible to the general public, as well as to scholars and students." Thus, the authors accomplish for Nightingale what she was unable to do for herself: edit her 829-page manuscript.

The editors' introduction to the abridged version of Nightingale's *Suggestions for Thought* places her writing in its biographical, historical, and philosophical context, providing readers with a succinct description of the religious and philosophical climate of the mid-Victorian era, and introduces many of the people and events that influenced Nightingale before she wrote *Suggestions*. The interaction between Nightingale and her famous contemporaries through correspondence and personal contact gives the reader fascinating insights into Victorian thinkers, reformers, and the Nightingale family.

The editors begin with "The Passionate Statistician," their description of Nightingale's passion for statistics. In "The Western Mystical Tradition," they then discuss her intellectual exploration, especially during her adolescence years, of Plato, Roman Catholic mystics, and select Eastern mystics. The editors suggest that the writing of *Suggestions* probably occurred while Nightingale was considering conversion to the Roman Catholic Church.

The next subtopics, "The Founder of Modern Nursing" and "The Struggle for Fulfillment," explore Nightingale's work in the context of her need to serve humanity and to practice nursing. The editors also suggest that the part of *Suggestions* referred to as "Cassandra" reflects Nightingale's struggle to find fulfillment as a single woman in Victorian England, and thus constitutes social criticism. I found Calabria and Macrae's references to Virginia Woolf and her knowledge of Nightingale particularly tantalizing and wished for further elaboration.

The introduction includes a brief discussion of Unitarianism and a review of influences from Germany and the East on Nightingale's writing. A lucent analysis of the Broad Church Movement in the Anglican Church follows, which makes a strong case for Nightingale's place in Broad Church thinking. The effect of evangelicalism and the general tone of religion in England are briefly

covered. Nightingale's problems with guilt and grace are identified but not explored.

The editors remind the readers that because Nightingale's piece was never a coherent, systematic book, but rather thoughts and reflections, their purpose was just to clarify her ideas and put them in a historical or biographical context. This is the strength of the volume.

The edited and abridged text of *Suggestions for Thought* includes her original dedication, and the seven chapter titles reflect the content: "On the Concept of God," "On Universal Law," "On God's Law and Human Will," "On Sin and Evil," "On Family Life," "On the Spiritual Life," and "On Life After Death."

The first four chapters appear to be Nightingale's attempts to explain her religious and philosophical beliefs. Some aspects of her thoughts are traced to early sources and some are not, probably to keep the volume from becoming cumbersome. For example, the editors comment that Nightingale rejected the doctrine of the atonement and believed instead that sin can only be driven away by learning from one's mistakes and that she was plagued by guilt. No additional explanation about atonement or guilt is included.

Nightingale may be at her best in the last three chapters on family and spiritual life. Anyone concerned with women's issues in general, as well as with nursing, will certainly find Nightingale's thoughts "On Family Life" important. The chapter "On Spiritual Life" is beautifully edited.

The hermeneutical framework Nightingale used to formulate her beliefs should be helpful to nurses who are seeking to describe and explain human phenomena. Indeed, I often found myself wishing to engage in discourse with Nightingale and sometimes the editors. They state their hope that their readers' minds will be stimulated from reading the book, and indeed the margins of my copy are filled with questions and comments for further reflection. Perhaps others will also find that this stimulating reading ignites such sparks.

Calabria and Macrae provide an excellent piece of scholarship in their treatment of Nightingale's *Suggestions*. They reveal the framework Nightingale used for her life and invite others to examine her thoughts as she matured. The book provides fertile ground for study and reflection by those interested in a glimpse into the inner life of a complex and productive woman.

JoAnn G. Widerquist, DMin, RN
Associate Professor Emirata
Saint Mary's College
Notre Dame, Ind.

And Sin No More: Social Policy and Unwed Mothers in Cleveland, 1855–1990

By Marian J. Morton
(Columbus: Ohio State University Press, 1993)

Noting that society has tended to look upon unwed mothers as unsympathetic and unworthy, Marian Morton in *And Sin No More* systematically uncovers the failings of private and public support for these women. Despite almost a century and a half of outdoor relief programs, institutionalization, the emergence of social work as a profession, and the medicalization of childbirth, support for these women remains inadequate. In fact, Morton suggests that social policy makers continue to label them as "unworthy" in order to provide them fewer services than the "deserving."

Morton's focus on Cleveland provides insight into the human effect of national policy as implemented at the local level. Tracing policy in one city allows the reader to understand the effects of changing demographics, norms, and markets on the client population.

And Sin No More is a multilayered study. On one level, Morton examines the plight of powerless women, whose problems were often compounded by poverty, traditional gender expectations, and race. She traces major themes in social policy, such as increased public accountability for health care and maintenance of dependent groups, and national trends, such as racial segregation and its decline, the women's movement, and the flight of Whites and the middle class out of the city.

Each chapter explores a different institution that provided care for unwed mothers during the study period and begins with a patient's admission or discharge notation. These poignant entries provide glimpses of the effects of policies on the lives of both dependents and providers. Perhaps more telling than the quotes themselves are the moral judgments made that controlled the allocation of health services to the women.

Chapter 1 examines the Cleveland Infirmary, the first institution for unwed mothers in the city. A patient register from 1856 lists the reason for admission as indigence brought about by "seduction." Institutionalization, although seen as less callous than outdoor relief, also allowed the agency to exert control over the lives of inmates through work and religious conversion.

Chapter 2 analyzes the Retreat, the Protestant effort to meet the needs of unwed mothers, which provided care from 1886 until 1936. The Retreat's goals were "spiritual conversion and physical reclamation." Chapter 3 examines the emergence of the social worker movement and its influence on private organizations. Redemptive maternity, requiring long confinement of unwed mothers with their infants, was contrary to social workers' desire for adoption, a less expensive and less time-consuming strategy.

Chapter 4 compares the institutional care given to unmarried rather than married mothers through the St. Ann's Infant and Maternity Asylum and its

subsidiaries from 1873 until 1983. In Chapter 5, Morton's examination of the Salvation Army's services for mothers based on marital status and race provides perhaps the most glaring examples of the inequities of policies made by one class for another. For example, policy makers established homes for White unwed mothers in far greater numbers than for Blacks, a practice based on stereotypical assumptions of the acceptability of unwed motherhood among Blacks.

Chapter 6, "Back to the Poorhouse," traces the cyclic outcome of inadequate support and conflicting policies for the unwed mother over time.

And Sin No More is an ambitious study of the consequences of social policy in one city across 135 years. Of special interest to social policy makers and historians, as well as health care providers and administrators, is Morton's ability to examine the care of unwed mothers within the larger context of power between those who formulate policy and those who are its recipients. Although the reader may perceive some redundancy across chapters, the real redundancy is the repetition of policies that produced inadequate services for a vulnerable and powerless population for over a century. Morton warns that America has been a society that allocates opportunities based on class, race, and gender and then punishes those who fail. At a time when public health care policy is being reformulated for all Americans, Morton's admonition is timely.

BONNIE L. RICHARDSON, PhD, RN
Assistant Professor
College of Nursing
University of Arkansas for Medical Sciences
Little Rock, Ark.

Bring Out Your Dead

By J. H. Powell
(Philadelphia: University of Pennsylvania Press, 1993; reprinted edition)

Reprinted on the 200th anniversary of the first major yellow fever epidemic in the United States, *Bring Out Your Dead* is J. H. Powell's sensitive recounting of the emergence and progression of this devastating disease and of the range of human behavior it provoked in the city of Philadelphia. A new introduction adds a contemporary perspective to the earlier preface and warns that yellow fever remains a potential threat.

Powell describes Philadelphia in 1793, then the national capital, as a crowded port city with a heterogeneous population of 55,000. One hot August Monday, physician Benjamin Rush diagnosed the first case of yellow fever, and by the end of the week, Philadelphia was in a shambles. As deaths and fears multiplied, thousands fled the city, and physicians debated whether the disease

was imported and contagious or domestic and carried through the air. People avoided one another, schools closed, businesses collapsed, the civic government fell into disarray, and Pennsylvania Hospital barred admission to anyone with yellow fever.

Lack of effective treatment and continuing mortality drove Rush to seek help in his medical books. Excited by the discovery of a yellow fever treatment to purge the body of "vicious humors," Rush relentlessly pursued a course of medical practice despite variable results and vigorous disputes about its efficacy with other physicians.

As yellow fever progressed, several leaders and a core of "common people" — among them Dr. Rush, the mayor, and a French-born merchant, Stephen Girard — began an organized resistance to the panic and miseries generated by the disease. Members of Philadelphia's Black community, for example, fulfilled many heroic and humane caregiving and burial roles. Other citizens settled disputes and served in hospitals and orphanages. Gradually, relief began to pour into the city from surrounding states.

Even though the epidemic peaked in October, melancholy pervaded the city and deaths continued unabated and without discrimination. Wealthy and prominent citizens, including physicians and the clergy, succumbed as rapidly as the impoverished and unknown. Cooler weather rekindled hope, but it was November before the number of daily deaths declined steadily and the city could begin its recovery and rebirth — although yellow fever was to strike again in subsequent years.

Two distinct but interrelated themes dominate Powell's account: health and disease during the early years of the United States, and human behavior in response to multiple stressors. Medical knowledge and treatment at the time were primitive, misguided, and often shocking, making disputes about causation and methods of care and cure inevitable. Powell's in-depth portrayal of Rush's efforts reveals how even an altruistic and dedicated physician often continued on an unproductive and dangerous path, and quietly confirms the value of peer review and standards for research that serve to negate the deleterious effects of self-deception and disregard for scientific caution.

Powell mentions nurses only as caretakers for the sick. But when eleven measures of prevention and protection were proposed by the College of Physicians, it was the first time in the new nation that government had asked a medical society for direction, perhaps an early signal of the need for an organized system of public health associated with local government.

Racial prejudice, professional exclusivity, and rigid nationalist sentiment among Philadelphians were not obliterated by yellow fever. It was easy to blame foreign refugees, like those recently arrived from Santo Domingo, for transmitting a new disease. Despite their significant service to the community, many Blacks were wrongly accused of profiteering and extortion, and the capable and intelligent medical efforts of foreign health care workers like French physician Jean Devèze generated consternation among local physicians.

Although Powell could not have foretold the current resurgence of infectious disease, he has provided ample enlightenment for contemporary profes-

sionals in all areas of health care. Physicians may take exception to the author's defense of Rush and become impatient with the primitive and often erroneous state of medical care 200 years ago, but there is much to be learned from the medical wisdom and pitfalls of the time. Nurse historians will note the scant recognition of nursing, but discerning readers will also detect examples of caring that have relevance for contemporary health care in general and nursing practice in particular. The book will also appeal to behaviorists and American history enthusiasts. Unique in its weaving of the timeless aspects of human behavior with an authentic account of a major epidemic in American and medical history, this book is carefully researched and a very good read.

GRACE P. ERICKSON, EdD, MPH, RNC
Assistant Professor
School of Nursing
Medical College of Virginia
Virginia Commonwealth University
Richmond, Va.

Cross Dressing, Sex, and Gender
By Vern L. Bullough and Bonnie Bullough
(Philadelphia: University of Pennsylvania Press, 1993)

This exhaustive work uses the specific topic of cross dressing to chronicle general issues of gender — including sexual identity, gender dysphoria, transvestism, and transsexualism — and to enumerate the multiple influences on gender-related attitudes and behavior. The book traces mythical and historical accounts of cross dressing from ancient to present times, relating various societal activities and specific cultural contexts to gender-related behavior.

The book's comprehensive approach permits the authors to examine the complexity of the phenomenon of cross dressing. The Bulloughs assert that prescribed gender roles differ in each culture and society. While gender is biologically determined, the authors posit that accepted gender-related behavior is wholly culturally determined, an assertion they support with many examples. The Bulloughs argue further that, in general, most societies have discounted individual differences in the definition of gender roles, a phenomenon they relate to the preponderance of male-dominated societies. Men, the authors point out, have less rigidly prescribed roles but more societal hostility toward deviation from those roles; women, on the other hand, have more rigidly determined roles but a more tolerant societal milieu.

The Bulloughs describe the ubiquitous nature of cross dressing as an expression of androgyny, supporting their case with examples from many cultures and religions. The authors illustrate their extensive discussion of esoteric Hindu

(and parallel Islamic and Buddhist) beliefs in the ideal of androgyny with examples from legend, worship, and culture. For example, Sardanapalus, the last of the Assyrian Kings, caused an uprising because of his practice of dressing as a woman. His subjects' revolt was based on their belief that cross dressing expressed weakness of character. In another illustration, the Egyptian princess Hatshepsut (fifteenth century B.C.) cross dressed because she felt limited as a leader by her gender. Her actions were seen by her people as a betrayal, and despite having served as an able leader, she was executed. These stories are meant to demonstrate the authors' belief that men cross dress for erotic pleasure, while women tend to cross dress to enjoy the greater freedom of males.

The authors also present a thorough discussion of gender and the arts, notably theater, where cross dressing has always been commonplace as a medium for social commentary. As early as the thirteenth century until well into the seventeenth century, men portrayed females on stage without social stigmas; the stage was generally described as "no place for a proper woman." As female actors became more common in the nineteenth and twentieth centuries, however, theatrical cross dressing evolved into "drag" acts.

In the years following World War II, transsexualism came under intense clinical scrutiny, and gender dysphoria became a focus of clinical medicine. The authors discuss the role of sexual reassignment in the sociology of gender—from the early surgical sex change experiences of Christine Jorgensen to current practice in medical centers worldwide—and relate evolving ideas of mental disorders concerning gender to social theory, all in the context of current attitudes toward sexual openness and expression. The phenomena of gender identity in twentieth-century America and the roles of twentieth-century theorists and professionals in defining gender issues as mental illness are discussed as well. Finally, the implications of cross dressing and transvestism are explored, and a chapter entitled "What to Do About Cross Dressing" is included. The volume contains a valuable postscript that could be published as a highly readable and comprehensive treatise on gender identity in societal context.

The audience for this book would certainly include those interested in gender and societal definitions of gender-related behavior. Painstakingly referenced and indexed, the book is a valuable resource for scholars and others interested in tracing gender-related phenomena through time. The book's later chapters, more easily understood by nonscholars, will prove especially valuable to mental health professionals working with patients needing support in gender identity issues and with families coping with cross dressing.

One possible weakness in this work is the Bulloughs' attempt to cover such a wide range of material. However, despite its broad scope, this book treats its issues thoroughly and makes an invaluable scholarly contribution.

MARY RAMOS, PHD, RN
Health Sciences Center
University of Virginia
Charlottesville, Va.

Educating for Health and Prevention: A History of the
Department of Community and Preventive Medicine of the
Woman's Medical College of Pennsylvania
By Bonnie Blustein
(Nantucket: Watson Publishing International, 1993)

Preventive medicine and community health have always been marginal in the
curricula of American medical schools, but some departments of preventive
medicine manage to ride the changing tides of medical thought and even to
flourish in the process. Blustein traces the history of one such program, the
Department of Community and Preventive Medicine (DCPM) in the Medical
College of Pennsylvania (formerly the Woman's Medical College of Pennsylvania), from the 1850s to the present.

From its inception, the Woman's Medical College of Pennsylvania was
committed to the teaching of preventive medicine and personal and public
hygiene, an interest that flowed from late-nineteenth-century advances in science and social reform. Classes in hygiene were based on the medical sciences of
physiology and bacteriology, as well as on the moral belief that whatever promoted the physical well-being of the individual and the community also promoted their moral well-being.

Dean Martha Tracy, an innovator in the field of preventive medicine, established the Department of Preventive Medicine at the College. By the 1940s,
however, advances in basic medical science and clinical practice led to severe
cuts in the curricular time allotted to preventive medicine. Following World
War II, leaders in the field joined forces to improve preventive medicine's image
by establishing a theoretical basis for the discipline. Their efforts were supported nationally by physicians who feared that unless their profession became
concerned with issues of prevention, a system of state medicine might be established.

In keeping with this trend, the Woman's Medical College appointed Kath-
arine Boucot Sturgis to chair its revitalized department. Sturgis added biostatis-
tics and public health to the curriculum, initiated research programs on the
prevention of pulmonary disease, and established clinical programs in occupational health and health maintenance. Ironically, renewed national interest in
preventive medicine led to a weakening of the department's strength, since
content on prevention was increasingly included in all medical specialty areas.

Social changes in the mid-1960s ushered in a new era for preventive medicine. However, DCPM practitioners often found their goals in conflict with
those of the racially segregated and polarized communities they hoped to serve.
Tension resulted when community residents perceived that the DCPM's initiatives were motivated more by a desire to provide experiences for medical students than to aid the community.

As federal funding disappeared, students became less socially active and
more focused on the curative aspects of medicine. The concept of prevention

was only tacitly accepted by the faculty, and the department again found itself in a peripheral position in the college. Learning from its past, the department revitalized itself through innovative curricular changes, shifting its focus to four distinct areas: occupational and environmental medicine, medical humanities (including bioethics), community health, and medical research design. These focuses came to be regarded as vital elements in the college's curriculum.

In a profession whose mission is the treatment of illness, what is the rationale for a specialty whose aim is the promotion of wellness, which, if successful, would eliminate clients' need for medical treatment? Is prevention common to all areas of medicine or is it a medical specialty with distinct subject matter? Faculty grappled with these and other issues during each stage of the DCPM's development.

Blustein asserts that the female character of the Woman's Medical College promoted its continuing emphasis on preventive medicine. Reflecting nine-teenth-century values that a woman's appropriate role was caring for family members, the founders of the college believed that female physicians in preven-tive medicine could combine the roles of scientist and domestic woman. Nine-teenth-century feminists argued that preventive medicine was a specialty for which women were particularly suited and one in which they could exercise their "moral superiority" for the benefit of society.

The book's major flaw is its omission of nursing. Although it mentions a preparation for "trained nurses" offered by the Woman's Medical College in the 1870s, only two other brief references appear.

The book should be of interest to nurse historians because of its examina-tion of an often unrecognized medical specialty. It also should be of interest to contemporary nurses who, during the present debate about national health care reform and the expanded roles of nurses, are assuming more independent roles as health care providers.

KAREN EGENES, EdD, RN
Assistant Professor
Department of Community, Mental Health and Administrative Nursing
Marcella Niehoff School of Nursing
Loyola University Chicago
Chicago, Ill.

The Healer's Tale: Transforming Medicine and Culture

By Sharon R. Kaufman
(Madison: University of Wisconsin Press, 1993)

The title says it all: society takes for granted that doctors heal; but because of changes within the discipline of medicine, society is now being forced to re-

assess important cultural questions, such as the meaning of curing, mother-hood, life, and death. To explain how and why this transformation is occur-ring, Sharon Kaufman, a medical anthropologist, interviewed seven retired physicians: Dunbar Shields, Saul Jarcho, Paul Beeson, Mary Olney, Jonathan Rhoads, Paul Hodgkinson, and John Romano. Their career histories provide the basis for Kaufman's thesis that contemporary Western medicine has manip-ulated nature, and in so doing has forced changes in our cultural beliefs about health and illness. This has resulted in moral confusion, the causes of which can be found in the medical profession's overreliance on technology—its devices, tools, and procedures—and its failure to inform society of the social worth of such technology.

Throughout the text, Kaufman intersperses selections from the interviews among her interpretation of the data. Using the doctors' remembrances of the 1920s and 1930s, she explores the prevailing medical morality and how physi-cians defined medicine and their roles at that period in history. All the doctors noted that they learned the meaning of duty and caring from their families. Medical training meant learning the "art of physical diagnosis" and the realiza-tion that many diseases could not be cured. In the 1920s and 1930s, medicine was in a period of continuity, and physicians had confidence in their skills and knowledge.

In the 1930s, at the beginning of specialization, the seven physicians started to combine clinical care with medical science. This process began with their residencies and continued with their assumption of academic teaching and scientific research roles.

In the 1930s and 1940s, the physicians speak of their sense of satisfaction as medical specialists. It was a period when experiments on live animals and pa-tients were acceptable for the advancement of science. Kaufman argues that during this era, medical morality—including the physicians' sense of responsi-bility, empathy, obligation, and respect for the patient and society as a whole—changed as medicine "embraced science" and became committed to the full use of technology and potent drugs in the curing of disease.

During the years between 1945 and 1965, when American medicine was at its zenith of prestige and political influence, the physicians considered the epit-ome of their medical careers to be their organizational work, with chief em-phasis still on responsibility to society and public service. Meanwhile, medical information and technology proliferated, medical centers and schools gained power and influence, clinical specialities developed subspecialities, and the de-livery of medical care began to become fragmented. At this point, a medical career, which for one doctor had been great fun and for another had offered limitless opportunities, began to change.

In her chapters on the 1970s to the 1990s, Kaufman explores the conse-quences of medicine's reliance on technology. She points out that specialists had succeeded in separating the individual into "body parts." Doctors had become unable to communicate satisfyingly with their patients, and the medical disci-pline was in a quandary with a public that on one hand expected medicine to be powerful and successful, but on the other hand challenged its authority and

expertise. Kaufman concludes that these "cultural effects" of medical practice have resulted in medicine losing its notion of the "shared good."

Besides Kaufman's main exposition on the transformation of medicine, this book has other strengths. The short biographies give the context of the medical careers of the seven physicians, and each recollection can be savored in and of itself.

However, I am left with several concerns. The recollections of the physicians have not been verified for historical accuracy. Kaufman has interpreted their statements to support her thesis; *they* did not speak of medicine's problems in terms of its "transformed identity." And though Kaufman argues that her sample is large enough to evaluate the culture of medicine from various perspectives, I remain skeptical that seven physicians can portray the U.S. medical profession.

Despite these problems, Kaufman is to be congratulated on her effort. She provides a focus for new dialogue on the health care system, a focus that will well serve nurse historians.

NATALIE N. RIEGLER, PhD, RN
Nursing Education Coordinator
Telemedicine Canada
Toronto, Ontario
Canada

Health and Medicine Among the Latter-Day Saints
By Lester E. Bush, Jr.
(New York: Crossroads Desk and Review, 1993)

One of a series of books examining human health practices within the context of the traditions of major religions, *Health and Medicine Among the Latter-Day Saints* introduces the reader to the beliefs and practices central to the Mormon way of life. Beginning with the emergence of Mormonism and the roles of founder Joseph Smith and his disciple Brigham Young, the author explores the conflicts generated by the introduction of a nonassimilated religion into a country that encourages assimilation. Of particular interest are the Americanization process that led to organizational changes within the structure of the religion, the establishment of behavioral standards within the church, and the implementation of an aggressive and highly successful missionary program extending throughout the world.

Organized into eight chapters, the book focuses on Mormon concepts basic to death and dying, wellness and suffering, healing, madness, sexuality and birth, morality and dignity, and caring. In the chapter on death and dying, the author discusses various Mormon beliefs, including those related to suicide, euthanasia, and burial rites. Acceptance of the Mormon concepts of death and

dying is germane to understanding the Mormon concept of the meaning of life. For example, many Mormon rituals, like baptism and purification, are believed to ensure eternal existence, and baptism of the dead by proxy makes salvation possible for ancestors. In fact, the importance of the search for ancestors is reflected in the strong emphasis on genealogy in the Church of Jesus Christ of the Latter-Day Saints.

The chapter on wellness and suffering demonstrates that health is valued in the Mormon tradition and is achieved through education, specific dietary restrictions, and avoidance of high-risk substances like alcohol, tobacco, and drugs. Suffering is seen as a natural consequence of disease and intrinsic to earthly existence.

The Mormon concept of healing centers on the historical role of the priesthood, the laying on of hands, anointing, prayer, and the use of herbs. Embedded in the religion itself, healing and faith are intertwined and encompass an alternative model to traditional medical practice. The church's gradual acceptance of modern medicine was not without conflict; in many instances, advances in modern science, medicine, and technology were antithetical to Mormon theology and accommodation was not easily attained.

With respect to madness, early Mormon thinking was rooted in the notion of devils and demons, which could be eliminated through religious rites performed by priests. These beliefs changed at the end of the nineteenth century with the acceptance of mental illness as a psychological phenomenon. Mormon treatment of mental illness at the time, according to the author, constituted a "gospel-based psychotherapy," a practice that, to some extent, survives today, but not without serious controversy among church officials.

The concept of caring, according to Mormon principles, is more a congregational endeavor than one associated with the helping professions. Thus, medical and nursing practice are given little consideration by the author in his discussion of the Mormon caring framework. An early Mormon church hospital system has since undergone divestiture to facilitate the church's involvement in international health-related activities.

The authority of the church is explicit throughout the book, and many early ideals and authoritarian principles have survived irrespective of changes over time. For example, Mormonism still espouses that individuals have a personal responsibility to maintain healthful practices. Church guidance is usually available on matters of personal concern and is based on current policies.

Health and Medicine Among the Latter-Day Saints is an introductory survey of Mormon beliefs and practices and is a potential resource for social scientists, anthropologists, and health care professionals seeking a beginning understanding of Mormon life. Although little attention is given to the specific role of nurses in the Mormon community, the book does provide information needed to make those services more relevant. In presenting his material, the author relies heavily on scriptural documentation and church publications and significantly less on historical interpretation. Several important content areas (e.g., caring and morality and dignity) lack adequate discussion and clarification, leaving the reader with many unanswered questions.

Despite its flaws, it is an interesting, informative, and readable book, which, according to the author, presents the first general publication of the Mormon Health Code and healing modalities.

NETTIE BIRNBACH, EdD, RN, FAAN
Professor Emeritus
Health Science Center at Brooklyn
State University of New York
Brooklyn, N.Y.

A History of Mental Health Nursing
By Peter Nolan
(London: Chapman & Hall, 1993)

Peter Nolan's excellent *A History of Mental Health Nursing* provides the first comprehensive analysis of the development of psychiatric nursing in Great Britain from its emergence in the middle of the nineteenth century to the present. Traditional histories of psychiatry, often written by psychiatrists, depict psychiatric care as an ongoing process of humanitarian enlightenment and scientific progress. Rarely, asserts Nolan, do these traditional histories of psychiatry acknowledge the experience and contribution of nurses. In fact, nurses — traditionally ranked in the middle and lower strata of the asylum hierarchy — are often stereotyped as indolent, unintelligent, and poorly qualified.

As part of the antipsychiatric movement of the 1960s, critical social theorists like Thomas Szasz, R. D. Laing, David Rothman, and the French philosopher Michel Foucault criticized the characterization of psychiatric care as enlightened. These critics depicted mental hospitals as institutions of social control or bourgeois repression, and emphasized that the history of psychiatric care has been largely limited to an account of the role psychiatrists have played within the movement.

Without taking sides in this debate, Nolan argues that the skepticism of the antipsychiatric movement empowered nurses to question the judgment made by many historians that psychiatric nurses have played only a marginal role in the history of care for the mentally ill. Using the perspective of social history and the context of contemporary social issues, Nolan seeks to help mental nursing find its own identity, separate from that of psychiatry, and to restore to it its rightful place in the history of mental health care.

A psychiatric nurse himself, Nolan is clearly motivated by sympathies for his profession and by a desire to contribute to its growth. The scope and range of Nolan's study are extensive; however, his historical condensation of mental health nursing has been accomplished at the expense of depth of analysis at some points.

Nolan reconstructs his history through both written sources and the oral

histories of nurses working in mental hospitals. He uses these invaluable materials to analyze the changing patterns of psychiatric nurse training and practice. Though its primary focus is nursing, the book also considers the contributions of psychiatrists to the establishment of psychiatric nursing, describing psychiatrists' influence and control over the training, employment, and practice of nurses.

Nolan begins his exploration with the care of the mentally ill prior to the asylum system. Initially employed as servants and workers on the asylums' farms, the first attendants were untrained. In late-nineteenth-century Britain, however, psychiatrists influenced by new ideas on moral therapy introduced formal training for mental health nurses that stressed new therapy and the moral conduct of the nurse.

Asylum overcrowding, the narrow focus of the mental nurses' training programs, and the difficult working conditions of the students and graduate nurses, however, prevented the desired improvements in patient care. Furthermore, the introduction of a formal mental health program outside the country's general nursing training system provoked strong reactions among nurse leaders. The result of these actions was that mental nurses were denied entry into British nursing organizations.

Nolan expertly uses nurses' personal accounts to illustrate their poor working conditions, low pay, and their growing activism to redress the inequities. Between 1930 and 1960, new therapies, including insulin, electroconvulsion, and drugs, as well as the introduction of psychotherapy and rehabilitative activities, slowly altered nurses' roles. Nolan points out, however, that although nurses played a central role in the management of mental institutions and served as the major source of guidance and comfort to patients, they rarely possessed the authority to define or control either patient care or their own working conditions. Not until the oppressive patient conditions in institutions became a matter of public debate were the nurses able to take some control over their own practice.

Using Hildegard Peplau's and Olga Church's analyses of the history of American psychiatric nursing, Nolan contrasts British mental nursing with that of the United States. He concludes that although there were similarities, American psychiatric nurses were more successful in creating independent identities and therapeutic roles than were British nurses.

Historically, Nolan notes, the care of the mentally ill has not only been difficult and demanding but has served as a constant source of disagreement among and between politicians and professionals. British nursing, however, is gaining more control over its education and practice, and the current shift from institutions to community care ensures that nursing will become more essential in the care of the mentally ill.

This well-researched book provides nurse historians and psychiatric nurses with a fascinating review of the British history of mental health nursing. Because of the dearth of historical knowledge about mental health nursing in Europe, Nolan's book makes a welcome contribution to psychiatric historiography. In addition, Nolan achieves his stated goal of providing psychiatric

nurses with a professional history that confirms the legitimacy of the services they provide.

GEERTJE BOSCHMA, MSN, RN
Doctoral Candidate
School of Nursing
University of Pennsylvania
Philadelphia, Pa.

Medicine and the Five Senses

Edited by W. F. Bynum and Roy Porter
(Cambridge, U.K.: Cambridge University Press, 1993)

Nurse educators, historians, theoreticians, and practitioners engaged in the quest for new knowledge, therapeutic effectiveness, and theories of practice will be interested in the questions addressed by the essays in *Medicine and the Five Senses*. How does the mind integrate the impressions generated by the five senses into some coherent whole? What role do sensory experience, intuition, and reason (considered to be the sixth sense) play in diagnosis? What should be the role of patients in diagnosing and determining their own therapy? Lastly, has technology diminished the therapeutic patient-nurse relationship?

Medical practitioners have always relied on a combination of reason, intuition, and sensory perception to diagnose and treat disease. The editors, social and intellectual historians of medicine and science, bring to the book's essays diverse perspectives on the development and conflicts in the use of the senses in the practice of medicine. Beginning with the ancient Greeks and extending into the present, the authors discuss the priority accorded to information gathered from the patient by the "noble" senses of vision and hearing and the "base" senses of touch, smell, and taste.

Medicine has sought, like Sherlock Holmes, to deduce the causes and treatment of disease from facts gathered by the physician. The physician-as-detective analogy in Vivian Nutton's essay "Galen at the Bedside: The Methods of a Medical Detective" argues persuasively that Galen was a practitioner who used the patient's information about his or her life, as well as information obtained through the physician's senses, to arrive at a diagnosis. Treatment consisted then of prescribing treatment and guiding adjustments in the patient's life to ensure recovery.

The reliance of medicine on the sense of interior vision, or consultation, has, on occasion, been detrimental to the patient. Roy Porter's essay "The Rise of Physical Examination" describes the last illness of the philosopher David Hume. For two months, Hume's physicians consulted with him and each other about the cause of his rapid physical decline, attributing it to a bilious complaint. It is obvious from Hume's writings that his physicians had "reasoned"

his diagnosis through history-taking and gross visual assessments, but had never physically examined their patient. As the result of a chance encounter between Hume and anatomist/surgeon John Hunter, the diagnosis of what was probably terminal cancer of the liver — a palpable liver tumor — was found. It is ironic that the demise of the philosopher most associated with antirationalism demonstrated the value of sensory experience.

Stanley Reiser's *Technology and the Senses in Twentieth-Century Medicine* argues that the diminishing confidence by both patient and physician in the use of the senses in diagnosis portends their limited role in the future of medicine. As imaging technologies, laboratory examinations, and computers have altered the diagnostic habits of physicians, the nature of the physician-client interaction has been drastically transformed. The computer and holograph can render the presence of both patient and physician unnecessary to the interaction. Patients and physicians (and their insurance companies) seek hard data, especially technologically based diagnostic tests, before accepting a diagnosis and treatment protocol.

The growing reliance on technology that focuses on physiological changes seriously minimizes the value of patients' description of how they feel and why they believe they may be ill. It also minimizes the value of physicians' clinical skills and talents and leaves them with a hermeneutic function, translating technological, interpreted data to their patients. The patients' personas, their narratives of how the illness affects their lives and mental states, and their roles in determining their own health care are threatened by the current technological revolution.

The essays in *Medicine and the Five Senses* assume that the senses and sensibilities of nurses play no significant role in the caring and curing of patients, and sources and accounts of nurses or nursing are scarcely referenced. However, the authors' well-illustrated studies and bibliographies offer opportunities for nurses to examine carefully the cogent questions posed by the book.

VIRGINIA M. DEFORGE, DNSc, RN
Associate Professor
Division of Nursing
Massachusetts College of Pharmacy and Allied Health Sciences
Boston, Mass.

Microbes and Minié Balls: An Annotated Bibliography of Civil War Medicine

By Frank R. Freemon
(Rutherford, N.J.: Fairleigh Dickinson University Press, 1993)

Named after the twin scourges that plagued doctors during the American Civil War, this comprehensive annotated bibliography of publications dealing with

medical care during that war is divided into primary and secondary sources. The primary sources include books and articles by Civil War doctors, nurses, and hospital attendants. Several diary entries by wounded, hospitalized, or imprisoned soldiers provide the perspective of contemporary health care recipients.

Secondary sources include not only materials that directly address Civil War medicine, but also those that touch upon medical care in general or that offer descriptions of the health of military and political leaders of the time. Important contemporary medical publications are annotated as well. Each annotation provides a basic subject overview and most are sufficiently detailed to assist readers in understanding the sources. The volume, which has an extensive index, also contains an alphabetized overview of Northern and Southern authors. Interestingly, Freemon encourages his readers to communicate to him any errors or oversights they might find in the book.

Freemon argues that the impact of the American Civil War cannot be fully grasped without an understanding of its medical history. His excerpts from primary sources lend insight into the art and science of medical practice at that time.

For example, in one wrenching episode, a Private Watkins — whom Freemon credits as the author of one of the best books written by a Confederate soldier — describes his visit to a wounded friend in the hospital. Pulling down the patient's blanket, Watkins discovers that the lower part of his body was mangled, with his entrails lying on the cot with him.

The book is comprehensive, containing references to official records of the Union and Confederate Navies, as well as the United States Sanitary Commission. Freemon annotates the twelve-volume series *The Medical and Surgical History of the War of the Rebellion* and Mary Livermore's *Numbers and Losses in the Civil War* (generally considered the definitive account of the dead, wounded, captured, and missing in the war's major battles), as well as three works by Samuel P. Moore, surgeon general of the Union Army, and four works by George Otis, who enumerated and summarized all operations performed during the war by surgeons on both sides of the conflict.

The book also refers to the works of many women authors, among them Southern nurses (Fannie Beers, Kate Cumming, Phoebe Yates Pember, Elvira Powers, and Susan Smith) and Northern nurses (Louisa May Alcott, Emily Elizabeth Parsons, Hanna Ropes, Adelaide Smith, and Amanda Stearns). Freemon annotates three of Florence Nightingale's works as well.

This gem of a book will be an invaluable aid to anyone engaged in historical inquiry of the Civil War and will appeal especially to those interested in Civil War medicine or nursing. Medical and nursing historians can use the bibliography to trace the development of the ambulance service, the hospital system, hospital ships, or the contributions of Black nurses and nuns during the Civil War. The bibliography also suggests future research that might focus on the war's "invisible enemies": infected wounds, poor nutrition, and poor sanitation.

Finally, the primary and secondary sources gathered in this bibliography invite analysis of some interesting historical questions regarding medical prac-

tice during the Civil War. How, for example, did the medical and nursing care received by the military during the war affect its outcome? Did Southern medical successes prolong the war or did Southern medical failures contribute to the South's ultimate defeat? The answers to these and other questions are made more possible by the book's extensive reference work.

MARIE E. POKORNY, PhD, RN
Associate Professor
School of Nursing
East Carolina University
Greenville, N.C.

The Nature of Suffering and the Goals of Medicine
By Eric Cassell
(Oxford: Oxford University Press, 1993)

The mysteries and nature of suffering and the relationship of suffering to the science and art of medicine enticed Cassell to write this thoughtful, historical book. Arguing that the obligation of physicians to relieve suffering stretches back to antiquity, Cassell explores the historical antecedents that shaped the shifting views of disease and the ideal physician. Identifying technology, objective science, and changes in the doctor-patient relationship as powerful factors in defining medicine, the author maintains that science, causality, and objective knowledge became the dominant values within the discipline. Asserting that the science and the morality of medicine are not opposed, Cassell urges physicians to recognize that it is *people* who suffer with and from diseases, and that it is the moral obligation of doctors to demonstrate devotion to the relief of *persons* suffering illness, rather than to focus solely on the cause and treatment of diseases. Hoping to revitalize medicine's moral perspective, Cassell urges physicians to move beyond the traditional dichotomy between mind and body, and to understand and internalize the concept of suffering.

Cassell devotes several chapters to explaining the nature of suffering and to illuminating its effects upon each aspect of personhood (the lived past, family, culture, roles, relationships, body, unconscious mind, perceived future, and the transcendent being). Cassell argues that while physicians are very concerned with the relief of pain or the restoration of lost function, these tasks result in one of the great paradoxes of medicine. That is, by virtue of their role in society to treat disease and restore function, physicians are obligated both to induce and to ameliorate suffering. In order to face suffering, Cassell urges physicians to overcome their fear of personal weakness and, as healers, to face the conflicts involved with patients' suffering.

Pointing out that disease affects the body's organs and molecules while illness afflicts the entire person's life, Cassell observes that the care of ill persons can only occur within the context of a relationship. He posits that the increasing

disregard and derogation of the doctor-patient relationship has created the erroneous belief that patients who are cured of disease are also healed.

Using vignettes, Cassell contrasts the pursuit and treatment of disease with the care and treatment of suffering persons in the context of their lives. He gently criticizes physicians' tendency to pursue "real" entities, like symptoms and disease, and urges them to move beyond the physical body to consider the lived experience of illness as the whole of a person's life. Arguing that all the manifestations of illness and suffering belong within the physician's domain, Cassell believes that the physician *is* the treatment, and that while this is the era of medical care teams, who support the physician, healing the whole person and alleviating his or her suffering is inherent in the physician's role.

While not a historical work, many of Cassell's ideas regarding the concepts of person and suffering offer historians interesting insights as they interpret the past. Nurses, both clinicians and historians, will not overlook Cassell's assertion that physicians "own" the healing relationship, the professional response to suffering, and the care of the whole person. While the book does exude a "captain of the ship" attitude and uses ideas that nurses have traditionally claimed, Cassell's argument highlights tenacious, unanswered questions regarding the nature of nursing; the conceptual boundaries between medicine and nursing; the meanings of such terms as *multidisciplinary, interdisciplinary,* and *transdisciplinary;* and the issue of who will pay for the time necessary for human understanding within a professional-patient relationship.

Cassell's book will appeal to readers who are interested in history, philosophy, ethics, the culture of the disciplines, suffering, and patient care. The book offers hope that by reexamining physicians' habits of thinking, being, and doing, the discipline of medicine will focus on ill people rather than diseases, thereby dissolving the boundary between cure and care.

DIANE HAMILTON, PhD, RN
Associate Professor of Nursing
School of Nursing
University of Rochester
Rochester, N.Y.

New Orleans' Charity Hospital: A Story of Physicians, Politics, and Poverty
By John Salvaggio
(Baton Rouge: Louisiana State University Press, 1993)

This history of New Orleans' Charity Hospital's 250-year struggle to serve the medical needs of the indigent poor is also a story of the physicians, politics, and patronage that either supported Charity or allowed it to deteriorate to the point of losing its accreditation.

The story begins with a description of the plight of slaves, early settlers, and other indigents who, though ill, were denied access to care at the Royal Hospital in New Orleans. Horrified by their ordeal, Jean Louis, a French seaman and ship builder, bequeathed his estate to the founding of Charity Hospital to care for the medical needs of the poor. Five Charity hospitals—the first constructed at Bienville in 1736—preceded the building of the current hospital in 1939. The early hospital was supported by a one-cent tax on slaves and on each acre of land. All admitted to the hospital provided work according to their abilities.

Salvaggio goes on to trace the evolution of the hospital and its care after Louisiana was ceded to Spain in 1763. For a time, monies obtained from taverns, bars, boarding houses, and fines were used to provide for the upkeep of the hospital. Under Spanish dominion, to practice medicine in the hospital, physicians—many of them still French—had to show a certificate of study, take an examination from the king's physician, and be a member of the Catholic church. All practitioners had to serve six months at the Charity or Royal Hospital without pay.

Subsequent chapters discuss the recurrent epidemics prevalent in the early settlements, the role of Charity Hospital during the Civil War, the management of the hospital by the Daughters of Charity, and medical education at the hospital. In 1895, under the supervision of Mary Agnes O'Donnell, a graduate of Bellevue Hospital School of Nursing, Charity's School of Nursing was established.

Most of the book focuses on the political problems confronting Charity Hospital during Governor Huey Long's era, the 1930s (when there were so many patients in the wards that they were often placed two in a bed), the post–World War II years, and the Earl Long period. Salvaggio also discusses extensively the trials and problems that arose in the 1970s—the infighting among members of the medical community and the administrative and medical nightmares of 1975 to 1980. Little changed at Charity during the 1980s, though the hospital appears to have received a reprieve in the 1990s, when it received a federal grant to construct a large Charity/LSU/Tulane–sponsored General Research Center within the hospital.

At the outset of the book, Salvaggio states that this work is a definitive history of Charity Hospital, but he offers limited information concerning the role nursing may have played in this drama. If nursing had no role, then the author should explain the reason for it. It would have been refreshing, and would have added something to the history, if representatives from the nursing staff had been interviewed as well as the physicians and hospital administrators.

Through an extensive review of political records, newspaper articles, interviews, important historical documents, and works of medical historians, Dr. Salvaggio does, however, weave a colorful and fascinating story of a hospital that was an integral part of New Orleans history for over two centuries. Throughout that time, Charity Hospital provided important leadership in medical care. This book, which contains many photographs of hospital wards in the early years, also points out in detail the role politics can play in the functioning and malfunctioning of a medical hospital. Historians, especially of institutional

history, should find this book an important source of information. Others will simply find it a fascinating history of people and events that shaped one of the country's well-known hospitals.

MYRTLE P. MATEJSKI, PhD, RN
Professor
College of Nursing
University of Delaware
Newark, Del.

William Henry Welch and the Heroic Age of Medicine

By Simon Flexner and James Flexner
(Baltimore: Johns Hopkins University Press, 1993; reprinted edition)

What health care analysts and policy makers frequently overlook in the current debate on health care reform is the role the American system of medical education has played in contributing to the current oversupply of medical specialists and to the undersupply of primary care practitioners. By emphasizing the research and scientific aspects of medical specialties, academic medicine encourages physicians to contribute to the expanding knowledge base of medicine rather than deliver primary care and preventive services. The recent reissue of Simon Flexner and James Flexner's 1941 biography, *William Henry Welch and the Heroic Age of Medicine,* sheds light on the evolution of the U.S. medical education system.

Dr. Welch, a bacteriologist and pathologist, was instrumental in developing the current system of medical education. The first dean of the Johns Hopkins Medical School, Welch was not only a theoretician, but an implementer with the political skill to transfer his ideas into action. He is credited with importing German research methods and incorporating them into U.S. medical education. As the foremost advocate of the modern public health movement, Welch was considered by President Hoover to be the greatest statesman in the field of public health.

Simon Flexner, a student, medical colleague, and lifetime friend of Welch, shared with him the philosophy that medicine is a science and that all medical students should be taught through the laboratory method and within a university school of medicine. Simon Flexner and his coauthor and son, historian James Flexner, produced this biography, which remains an excellent account of Welch's life. By documenting the changing of American medicine into a research-based practice, this book offers important insights into today's crisis involving the delivery of medical care.

Adamant that medical students should learn about disease through laboratory observations, their own experimentation, and questioning rather than relying on the rote memorization of medical lectures, Welch demonstrated that the basic sciences were critical to the advancement of scientific medicine. In re-

sponse to the argument that this type of medical education would only produce teachers and researchers, Welch responded that the scientific habits of discipline and intellectual reasoning allowed all physicians a more astute way of dealing with patients' medical problems.

Under Welch's deanship, the Hopkins medical school adopted high standards for admissions and encouraged more faculty time spent on teaching and research by instituting a system in which medical faculty would be salaried. New to America, this practice freed the faculty from relying on a busy outside practice. Despite controversy surrounding this policy, Welch's charismatic leadership attracted many scientific notables to Hopkins. The chapter "Health of the Nation" provides a comprehensive, historically accurate account of Welch's activities in the field of publication, for which he is often best remembered. Nationally and internationally, he spoke for the scientific teaching of hygiene, a commitment reflecting his belief that no social, industrial, or economic problems existed that were not related to the problems of health.

Welch's interest in bacteriology ranged from laboratory research on diphtheria to the organizion and presidency of the National Association for the Study and Prevention of Tuberculosis. His influence ranged from the local, as a life-long member of the Maryland Board of Health, to the national, as an advisor to Theodore Roosevelt on the control of yellow fever in Panama, to the international, as the carrier of the message of modern scientific medicine to the Peiping Union Medical College in China.

The book's journey through William Welch's life is supplemented by fifty-six pages of text notes. Introducing hundreds of Welch's teachers, coworkers, family members, and friends, the book is truly a Who's Who of the scientists and statesmen of the Progressive Era and the Gilded Age. The biography represents almost a decade of research into a significant period in the history of American medical education, public health, and the development of the medical care system. Unfortunately, although nurse historians have noted Welch's staunch friendship with public health nursing, little about it is written in the Flexners' book.

This almost lovingly written account of one of America's most prominent physicians, who began his career almost a hundred years ago, is worthy of the attention of a new generation of readers. Those interested in the history of medicine, nursing, and public health will benefit from its extensive bibliography. In addition, the nursing profession might learn from medicine's total acceptance of the research model, and so proceed cautiously in its own quest for a research base for nursing. Finally, scholars of social and educational history will be challenged by the process of change that this biography explores.

ALICE H. FRIEDMAN, RN, MSN
Professor Emeritus
School of Nursing
University of Massachusetts
Amherst, Mass.

Birth as an American Rite of Passage
By Robbie E. Davis-Floyd
(Berkeley: University of California Press, 1992)

To what extent are current obstetrical protocols shaped by society's views of accepted childbirth? Robbie Davis-Floyd explores this issue by interviewing 100 middle-class American women about their birth experiences. The majority of these women described how they were hooked up to fetal monitors, had intravenous needles inserted into their arms, were given pitocin to augment their labor, and then received episiotomies. Interestingly, Davis-Floyd discovered that despite the feminists' harsh critique of such standard obstetrical interventions, most of the women interviewed found these practices not only acceptable but right.

Using an anthropological context, Davis-Floyd discusses the pregnancy-birth continuum as a year-long rite of passage for the mother, with pregnancy and childbirth constituting a transformation period during which she integrates society's norms and expectations. Relying on the metaphor of the body as a machine, Davis-Floyd points out that medical rituals and rites treat a woman's pregnancy and birth in a mechanistic manner. Pregnancy is seen as creating flaws in the "machinery" of a woman's body, prompting obstetricians to discover new and better ways to "fix" those mechanical problems. Davis-Floyd charges that childbirth is one experience that challenged twentieth-century culture to develop mechanical ways of dealing with a powerful natural and supernatural life experience. In accepting this view, however, society is confounded by the fact that babies are born of women, not machines, and no matter how we attempt to control the natural act of birthing, it remains uncontrolled.

The involvement of male partners in the birthing process is also explored by the author. Although the hospital's tolerance for men in the labor rooms has improved, 91 percent of the women interviewed were separated from their partners during such procedures as the "prep." Davis-Floyd argues that incorporating the partner into the labor and delivery experience is a new strategy by which the hospital can co-opt him into believing in the technocratic model. The author also believes that other labor and delivery ritual elements — such as beds, gowns, monitors, and Apgar scores — communicate symbolic messages about our culture's beliefs that nature is untrustworthy, female bodies are inferior, patriarchy is valid, science and technology are superior, and institutions and machines are essential.

The author presents two other models for interpreting pregnancy and childbirth — the holistic and the natural — both of which strongly contradict the prevailing technocratic models of hospitals. Davis-Floyd suggests that the rites and rituals of childbirth embraced by our current society are deeply embedded and, as such, will continue to view holistic or natural models of childbirth as unnatural. From interviews with twelve obstetricians, Davis-Floyd also discovered that the technocratic model is perpetuated through the socialization of physicians themselves in medical schools.

Only fifteen of the women interviewed actually desired and achieved natural childbirth in the hospital. Many received an especially high degree of medical intervention with their first births and were unable for almost a year to verbalize their feelings of grief, rage, and psychological anguish over their hospital treatment. For their second births, these women reported being better prepared to handle the medical method of childbirth and permitted fewer medical interventions.

The author admits that her own belief that childbirth rituals are medically and psychologically damaging to women made it difficult for her to understand how American women could accept the technocratic birth model. Indeed, Davis-Floyd's interviews revealed that many of the women found the technocratic interventions empowering. The author concludes that a woman's ultimate perception of her birth experience as positive or negative, empowering or victimizing, depends on the degree to which the experience confirms or undermines the belief system she brings to the hospital. According to the author, society's inability to indoctrinate every woman to accept without question the technocratic model of childbirth is a positive sign, because ideological diversity enhances a culture's ability to adapt to environmental changes.

This book will appeal to a wide range of readers, including historians, health care professionals, and consumers curious about obstetrical history and the medicalization of childbirth. In addition, the accurate depiction of the technocratic model of the 1980s presented in this book will offer future historians a view of the beliefs, values, rites, and rituals Americans now possess about childbirth.

PEGGE L. BELL, PhD, RN
Assistant Professor
College of Nursing
University of Arkansas for Medical Sciences
Little Rock, Ark.

Courage Under Siege: Starvation, Disease, and Death in the Warsaw Ghetto
By Charles G. Roland
(New York: Oxford University Press, 1992)

Historians of the holocaust have a distinct advantage in their work in that this event is at once both inherently gripping and inconceivable. However, because the events associated with the Holocaust have been the subject of such extensive research and writing in both scholarly and popular domains, there exists a challenge to approach inquiry from a new angle. An even greater challenge is to do so in a way that captures the sensationalism of the Holocaust without being sensational in writing about it.

Charles Roland meets both of these challenges successfully in his book *Courage Under Siege* through his study of the medical system that operated within the squalid confines of the Warsaw ghetto. Although the medical institutions and the underground medical school that operated in the ghetto form the centerpiece of the book, Roland effectively captures a significant portion of ghetto life as a whole, a life characterized by a constant, consuming struggle for survival against severe medical traumas — starvation, rampant communicable diseases, and injury. Roland's emphasis on the ghetto medical system not only makes an important contribution to understanding this less frequently studied aspect of ghetto life, but provides a valid perspective on the whole of ghetto existence.

Roland provides in his introduction an effective overview of the book's purpose: to describe the tradition and destruction of Jewish medicine in Warsaw, and to tell the story of the ghetto as medical history. The result is a report that grips the reader with its imagery and vivid realism.

The first three chapters provide a detailed discussion of Jewish medicine, the Nazi occupation of Poland, and the establishment of the ghetto itself. Remarkably concise, this discussion sets the stage for the focus on the medical system that follows. Even the uninformed reader receives sufficient background information to grasp the more intensive discussion of medicine and disease in the ghetto that occupies the majority of the text. Medical systems have historically been inextricably linked with broader social and political forces, and the Warsaw ghetto was no exception. Roland does a thorough job portraying the military and political forces that converged in the establishment of the ghetto and in the medical system itself, with its own awkward blend of successes and abuses.

The medical system of the Warsaw ghetto represents many of the brutal ironies associated with the lives of its residents. The Czyste hospital, for example, which formed the centerpiece of the ghetto medical system, deteriorated from what was considered a modern hospital of the 1930s to a place where patients died from hunger as well as from disease. Although nurses are noted as being actively engaged in care, nothing more is said of their presence.

One branch of the hospital ultimately became a shelter for Jews as they waited to board the cattle cars bound for Treblinka. Physicians often were called upon to make the "selection" — not only among patients but often among their own staff as well. These ironies, along with various other acts that can only be described as barbaric, are presented clearly and personally through Roland's story of the medical system.

The book's title refers to courage as well as to siege, and Roland offers substantial instances of it: the care provided by medical personnel against insurmountable odds, for example, and the students of a clandestine medical school who were forced to make the extremely dangerous trip to its building across ghetto boundaries. Roland also describes the rigorous research by physicians into the effects of starvation in an effort to have something positive come out of a helpless situation. Nonetheless, these acts of courage are often overshadowed by accounts of rampant disease and squalor. Ultimately, the courage and main-

tenance of life became secondary to the destruction associated with ghetto life and the Holocaust.

Overall, Roland has made a unique and highly credible contribution to the historical literature on the Holocaust. The book is extensively referenced with citations to a variety of archival materials, primary literature, and autobiographical sources, as well as to personal interviews conducted by the author. Also to Roland's credit, he directly confronts conflicts that exist in competing accounts of some events and offers explanations when reasonable. Although this is a scholarly book, the resulting text is concise and tightly integrated, reading much like a novella. While historians of the Holocaust, Judaica, and medical history will find that this book provides new insights and detail, it is compelling and provocative reading for all who consider themselves students of humanity.

BETH L. RODGERS, PhD, RN
Associate Professor
School of Nursing
University of Wisconsin-Milwaukee
Milwaukee, Wis.

Deviance and Medicalization: From Badness to Sickness
By Peter Conrad and Joseph W. Schneider
(Philadelphia: Temple University Press, 1992; republication)

When first published in 1980, this book won praise, awards, and an influential place among texts exploring the sociology of deviance. Its importance lay in its use of history to explain how and why increasing forms of problematic behaviors came to be defined as medical "diseases" and, hence, were proper subjects of medicine's own brand of social control. Conrad and Schneider approached the "disease" designations of mental illness, alcoholism, opiate addiction, homosexuality, criminality, and childhood delinquency, hyperactivity, and abuse as essentially political social constructions applied to powerless and subordinate people by powerful and influential interests. The historical reconstruction of deviance, they concede, with its conceptualization of the "sick role," has contributed a more humanitarian cast to the stigmatization of those judged to be different, and its interventions have created a more flexible, efficient, informal, and individualized form of control than that of our judicial and legal systems. However, they conclude, a more pernicious problem remains embedded within such seeming benevolence. The medicalization of deviance focuses on the individual and ignores the structure of the social system that shapes both the meaning and the expression of problematic behavior. Thus, in the final analysis, medicine acts as a de facto agent of dominant political interests and as a seemingly neutral scientific and expert embodiment of social control.

A decade ago, this thesis broke new conceptual ground in history, sociology, and related disciplines. In its 1992 republication, however, it seems flat, heavy-handed, and as reductionistic as the formulations it sought to replace. For while historians of health care can now no longer risk ignoring the ways in which medicine and nursing acted as agents of bourgeois social values, neither can they now risk ignoring the very real, positive differences these disciplines made in the lives of their patients and their communities. Many historians have moved beyond the social control theory per se to ask of their data, How did clinicians negotiate the dilemma of both caring for and controlling their patients (a dilemma, it must be pointed out, first faced by nurses as they gradually assumed the roles and responsibilities once under the dominion of the family)? Conrad and Schneider, however, have not moved beyond their original conclusion.

In a chapter on mental illness, for example, the authors argue that it is doubtful that madness is mental illness or even a medical problem, and presume that there has never been either physiological "evidence" or successful "medical" treatments that might justify a "scientific" disease model. Imagine the surprise of eighteenth- and nineteenth-century physicians and families who, as we now know, never constructed the authors' boundary between social and medical ideas about madness and its treatment. Families, especially, moved quite easily between the two in their quest to find some relief for themselves and for their kin.

It may be considered unfair to judge a 1980 work in the context of more recent scholarship except that Conrad and Schneider state "that new studies would not lead us to alter fundamentally our basic arguments and analysis." They do, however, address other critiques of *Deviance and Medicalization* — for example, the charge of "medical imperialism" (that is, the illegitimate medicalization of the social world when there is little evidence of power at the level of what physicians actually control and do) and the criticism of "ontological gerrymandering" (allowing commentators a privileged place from which to observe the "truth" of a social construction without attending to the social construction of their own analysis). Not even sociologists, they conclude, are immune to the wish to view their "scientific" practice as disinterested, or themselves as shorn of the desire for a more secure place in the intellectual deployment of power.

This last critique contains an important insight for historians of nursing. While theory remains the single most important tool for gleaning new insights from old data, theorizing itself is not without the pitfall of presentism. If this book does have value to scholars working today, it may be as a reminder that the pose of objectivity might be as much a social construct as the phenomena under study. This does not suggest abandoning the historical quest to understand the ideas and practices of our predecessors "on their own terms." One only needs to pay closer attention to the ways in which our own values and conceptualizations of nursing inevitably color our analyses of the past.

PATRICIA D'ANTONIO, PhD, RN
Merion, Pa.

The Evolution of Cardiac Surgery

By Harris B. Shumacker, Jr.
(Indianapolis: Indiana University Press, 1992)

Dr. Shumacker's comprehensive history on cardiac surgery can be read on two levels. First, it is a thorough, humane review of a specialized medical field that has changed the lives of many and helped reinforce the aura of the godlike surgeon. Second, the book is also the author's caring tribute to men he studied or worked with over a career that spanned more than half a century.

Dr. Shumacker is not an inexperienced writer who turned to publishing historical books in his retirement. *The Evolution of Cardiac Surgery* is his fifth historical work. He has published the histories of two medical societies, a biography of thoracic surgeon Leo Eloesser, and a biography of Dr. John Gibbon, who performed the first successful heart-lung machine–assisted cardiac surgery.

The book's contents follow the development of cardiac surgery from the first operative drainage of the pericardium to relieve the symptoms of constrictive pericarditis in the eighteenth century to the current practices of left ventricular devices and artificial hearts.

The author describes Greek and Roman views of the heart, including its place in art, and gives the reader an appreciation for the importance the heart has played throughout history. The book's chapter titles are organized by surgical procedure, such as "Coartaction Is Conquered," "Mitral Stenosis Revisited," and "Further Development of Heart-Lung Machines." Dr. Shumacker feels the contemporary period lasted from the late thirties, when surgeons could operate on congenital malformations and adjacent cardiac vessels, until 6 May 1953, when Dr. Gibbon ushered in the current era with his triumphant use of a heart-lung machine. Deep hypothermia, induced cardiac arrest, valve replacements, assist devices, and heart transplants all followed. Dr. Shumacker witnessed many of these advances, which occurred in the fortunate time before resource allocations, complex ethical dilemmas, and shrinking research monies.

Dr. Shumacker reveals a gee-whiz attitude toward his profession; he considers the evolution of cardiac surgery to be a "miracle." He is, of course, correct. The pace of discovery and advancement in cardiac surgery mirrored other technology in the twentieth century. In less than one hundred years, surgeons accomplished what their predecessors only imagined. Dr. Shumacker's enthusiasm also translates into a very readable history. There are no boring recitations of dates and facts in his book. He describes procedures, but we also learn about the patients themselves, like the twenty-two-year-old man who had been cut in the chest and who received pioneering pericardial repair in 1891. Such details help to humanize this sterile, scientific field. The reader also learns more about famous surgeons besides their names. For example, Alfred Blalock and his colleague Helen Taussig, whose names many nurses become familiar with during their parent-child nursing courses, decided to treat "blue babies" with tetralogy of Fallot by operatively creating a pulmonary-systemic shunt after they noticed that the babies did not become cyanotic until their ductus arteriosus closed.

Portrait photographs appear throughout the book, personalizing names and accomplishments. They also remind the readers how exclusive this White-male-dominated world was. A weakness in this book is that the reader is left with the impression that these surgeons worked alone. There is no mention of a surgical team, and the nursing profession is reduced to a minor role. Another history of this era that included the perspectives and contributions of nurses and other personnel who participated in these ground-breaking surgeries would provide a balance to Dr. Shumacker's book. So would an analysis of the aura that developed around these physicians.

Dr. Shumacker writes with a surgeon's knowledge. The surgical language he uses will make this book appealing to operating-room nurses. Historians will appreciate his use of context, including what knowledge surgeons possessed and what they accomplished with tools like sterile gloves and blood transfusions. His primary references are exhaustive but clearly presented in chapter notes. Anyone studying cardiac surgery will find these references excellent resources in themselves.

This book provides a reassuring glance of what an important contribution cardiac surgeons have made to society. Dr. Shumacker's book is a well-written history by a person who participated in the progress and successes of cardiac surgery.

ELIZABETH M. NORMAN, PhD, RN, FAAN
Associate Professor
College of Nursing
Rutgers, The State University of New Jersey
Newark, N.J.

The Evolution of Women's Asylums Since 1500: From Refuges for Ex-Prostitutes to Shelters for Battered Women

By Sherrill Cohen
(New York: Oxford University Press, 1992)

Sherrill Cohen suggests that as far back as the fifteenth century the response of society to those anomalous women it considers "out of place" has been an institutional one. Focusing primarily on the sixteenth through eighteenth centuries, Cohen uses the historical records of three convents or asylums for women to explore the social and historical significance of these early "refuges" for women and to draw parallels between these early institutions and a number of other institutional prototypes, including girl's schools, women's prisons and residences, homes for unwed mothers, and shelters for battered women. Though Cohen pointedly justifies her presentist approach, linking past and present, nearly all the connections between past and present are left to a concluding chapter.

The asylums whose records form the center of this book were founded by Catholic reformers in separate areas of Tuscany: the Monastero delle Convertite, a convent for penitent prostitutes; the Casa delle Malmaritate, which specialized in helping married prostitutes and other "troubled married women"; and Santa Maria Maddalena, a community of ex-prostitutes that eventually developed into a traditional cloistered convent. With little primary source material available from the residents of these convents, Cohen reconstructs life in them by examining institutional statutes and constitutions, administrative and financial records, and magisterial and police accounts.

Cohen does an excellent job of piecing together available data to highlight medieval and early modern gender ideology, the problem of prostitution, the rationale behind the operations of the three convents, and the social significance of the convents within the contexts of the local community and early modern society. The book emphasizes both the social context underlying the development of the convents and the day-to-day life within the institutions. For example, Cohen explores the apparent contradiction between the convent's promise of a "secure haven" and the punitive role of each institution. Rescue and punishment were often separated in early modern society by a fine line, the result of a gender ideology that portrayed women as both transgressors and victims. Thus, while some women were coerced into becoming nuns because they broke the rules governing prostitution, the path toward religious life also offered shelter for women who only wished to escape the insecurities of outside life. Marriage, seen as the optimal rehabilitation for prostitutes as well as the ultimate solution to concerns about insecurity, provided the primary way out of these institutions.

But only some women sought to leave. For others, institutional life presented the best of an extremely narrow range of alternatives, providing opportunities otherwise unavailable to many women in the world outside. For instance, residents had the chance to become literate and within certain limits to find opportunities for creative expression. Some residents seized economic advantages by speculating in investment funds called *monti* and accumulating property. Residents also played an active role in administering the institutions. Options were still limited, however, and societal norms intruded in numerous ways, such as the creation of a hierarchical arrangement, assigning lower status *servigiale,* or domestic nuns, to attend to the needs of higher status *velata,* or veiled nuns. But Cohen's evidence suggests that in the all-female convent communities, women actively sought ways to expand individual opportunities while trying new approaches to managing collective affairs.

As noted earlier, most of the presentist implications of this work are reserved for a single chapter, primarily an overview of the social legacies of early modern women's asylums. This may satisfy historians whose main interest is the case studies themselves, but will disappoint those for whom the title suggests a narrative more closely intertwining past and present. Cohen sees early women's asylums as the forerunners of a wide range of institutions, from men's and women's penitentiaries to maternity homes. Yet the examination of specific links is isolated and brief, resulting in tenuous conclusions. I was particularly disappointed to find only fleeting reference to schools of nursing and mental hospi-

tals; even the relationship to battered women's shelters is compressed to just over two pages that highlight parallels between medieval references to unhappy wives and the contemporary view that "residence in a battered women's shelter is . . . a path toward divorce" (p. 162).

Though Cohen's study suggests a historical tendency to institutionalize women in order to solve their problems, the book falls short of providing authoritative proof. Still, this book issues a meaningful challenge to scholars of social institutions who have generally regarded the sociopolitical development of institutions as essentially a modern innovation. Others, including students of early modern Europe and women's history, are also likely to find useful insights. In short, *Women's Asylums* provides intriguing case studies and suggests the need for expanded research into the evolution of social institutions, but it falters in its attempt to move from sixteenth-century Italian convents to contemporary shelters for battered women.

Tom Olson, PhD, RN
Assistant Professor
School of Nursing
University of Hawaii at Manoa
Honolulu, Hawaii

Mental Machinery: The Origins and Consequences of Psychological Ideas, 1600–1850

By Graham Richards
(Baltimore: Johns Hopkins University Press, 1992)

Graham Richards maintains that the invention of the discipline of psychology has been a more profound and complicated process than has been suggested by its historians. Richards, a self-professed Wittgensteinian, conceptualizes the invention of psychology as a linguistic process whereby psychological ideas were generated in a social-political-theological context during the period immediately preceding the recognition of psychology as a separate discipline (1600–1850). That is, rather than supporting the traditional historical view of psychology as a *discipline,* Richards has written a history of psychology as *subject matter* with the intent of emphasizing our failure to understand how thinkers *created* rather than *discovered* the inner realm of mental machinery.

Richards divides his book into three parts: the first section analyzes the content and motivation behind seventeenth-century thinking, the second explores the philosophical ideas and social context of the eighteenth century, and the third examines not only the distinctive German, British, and French social and psychological processes, but also the philosophy of language assumptions that eventually led to the collective endorsement of ideas that created the inner and public realms of psychology.

Richards's analysis of the language of speakers and listeners, as well as of

the linguistic content of speech and its meaning, begins with the canonical texts of Descartes, Hobbes, Locke, Hume, Mill, and others, with the aim of disclosing both the conditions under which the texts' ideas were produced and the issues they were intended to address. Richards argues that these early works transformed the view of the nature of man as a fixed universal entity in nature to a view of man as a dynamic individual capable of both a private vision of the world and individual perfectibility.

Drawing from the work of Michel Foucault, Andrew Scull, Vieda Skultans, Roy Porter, Kurt Danziger, and Steven Shapin, Richards analyzes the impact of technological, physiological, educational, sexual, and social role shifts upon psychological thinking, and moves beyond the social context of language to tease out and analyze the linguistic philosophic conditions that governed the possibility of generating new psychological ideas. This approach explicates how language became a vehicle of creative power that mediated between the human soul and God. Language, then, was not simply a transparent representation of thoughts, but had its own prophetic power, which became a route for exploring the psyche and perfecting mankind and his social world.

According to Richards, a psychological vocabulary made it possible to create a *mentality* that permitted the idea that the "inside" of man (the mind/soul) could be externalized, mechanized, and manipulated according to rational principles that would guide how life should be experienced and responded to. The scientific worldview became the touchstone of sanity, and the social role of the scientist became the epitome of the ideal person.

In conclusion, Richards argues that the creation of psychology and its agent, the psychologist, was a social process as much as it was a psychological one; it created a language and it created the collective social construction of new roles and the endorsement of their meanings. Richards's work demonstrates that the processes of signification are bound up with interpretations of texts and their context. By undercutting the dichotomy between text and context, Richards offers a rich metahistory of the development of psychological language as a precursor to the discipline of psychology. While a fascinating study, by the author's own admission the book is tortuous, its complexity and level of specialization recommending it neither to the passive nor the intellectually cowardly reader. This is a book written for historians who are either well-versed in or committed to understanding the post-Kuhnian methodological and linguistic debates involved within interdisciplinary studies (e.g., Hayden White and Ludwig Wittgenstein). Despite its denseness, the book offers important insights for nursing historians regarding the evolution of the metaphorical construct we have come to call nursing.

DIANE HAMILTON, PhD, RN
Assistant Professor
School of Nursing
University of Rochester
Rochester, N.Y.

Mortal Presidency: Illness and Anguish in the White House

By Robert E. Gilbert

(New York: Basic Books, 1992)

Gilbert's *Mortal Presidency* reinforces the thesis that all human beings, including presidents, are subject to the impact of stress and illness. Through a sobering historical record, he documents the debilitating medical problems, physical and psychological, that have profoundly affected the lives and administrations of U.S. presidents.

A general introduction describes the unique demands of the office of the president, which mandate that presidential health, disability, and mortality receive greater attention than ever before. Statistics in the form of actuarial tables are presented as evidence that twenty-five of our presidents have died prematurely, four of them by assassination. Even more surprising is the fact that those presidents who have lived the longest (beyond their life expectancy) were the first ten to hold office. The implications of these findings are significant, particularly since disability was for all practical purposes not recognized or addressed in the Constitution. Thus, in his final chapter, "Prescriptions," Gilbert analyzes the Twenty-fifth Amendment on presidential disability and succession. Among his recommendations is a plea that the vice presidency be upgraded and filled by individuals of presidential stature.

Perhaps the most interesting sections of the book for most readers will be the case studies of five twentieth-century presidents — Calvin Coolidge, Franklin Delano Roosevelt, Dwight Eisenhower, John Kennedy, and Ronald Reagan. Gilbert provides a medical profile for each of these presidents and examines the political effects of their illnesses. He probes their formative years as well as their time in office in order to construct a psychological profile that could potentially account for each president's vulnerabilities and the subsequent impact of these on governing ability.

The story of Calvin Coolidge is possibly the least familiar, yet the most poignant. His political effectiveness was literally destroyed by a deep depression resulting from the accidental death of his second son in 1924. Coolidge never recovered from his grief and essentially retreated from his executive responsibilities. In striking contrast, however, Gilbert portrays Franklin Roosevelt as a person who coped extremely well with polio and other medical problems while carrying out his responsibilities to the very end. John Kennedy is distinguished by "strength of character," a byproduct of his painful physical problems. According to Gilbert, no existing evidence suggests that physical problems or medications negatively affected Kennedy's presidency.

Some may question Gilbert's assumptions about Eisenhower and Reagan. Eisenhower suffered from a number of debilitating medical problems, including a heart attack and a stroke. Gilbert postulates that although Eisenhower's position of power exacerbated his ailments, he accepted the physical and emotional stresses as punishment for losing his mother's approval and love. In addition, Eisenhower felt responsible for the death of a son, which he also

considered a personal failure of duty. Gilbert speaks of repeated instances of self-destructive behavior in which Eisenhower "ignored reason" and chose to follow a more dangerous course, thereby risking physical calamity. In the case of Reagan, Gilbert asserts that he was psychologically vulnerable; he was an adult child of an alcoholic parent and tried to escape from the "black curse" of that addiction. According to Gilbert, this fact, as well as the 1981 assassination attempt and his cancer surgery in 1985, contributed to his denial of the Iran-Contra scandal and greatly affected his administration.

Although historians may wish that more rigorous methods had been followed, psychologists may believe that the psychological profiles are too superficial, and politicians may feel that the book adds little to the continual debate about reforming the American presidency, Gilbert raises interesting questions worthy of consideration by anyone, especially nurses and nurse historians. This book would be particularly useful in an issues course, since it touches on and illustrates the complexity of all aspects of society — sociology, politics, psychology, economics, ethics, and even religion.

M. PATRICIA DONAHUE, PHD, RN, FAAN
College of Nursing
University of Iowa
Iowa City, Iowa

Philanthropy and the Hospitals of London: The King's Fund, 1897–1990
By F. K. Prochaska
(Oxford: Clarendon Press, 1992)

This book, a thorough and intricate account of the origin and evolution of the King's Fund — launched by Edward, Prince of Wales (later King Edward VII), at the time of Queen Victoria's Diamond Jubilee in 1897 — represents a landmark in the British literature about philanthropy, charities, the voluntary hospital system, the state health system, and the emergence of the modern hospital. The first comprehensive treatment of the role of the King's Fund, this work challenges numerous interpretations of hospital provision in Britain in terms of the broader issues of the history of social policy.

Prochaska establishes the context out of which the Fund emerged: the efforts of those who sought to rescue the impoverished hospitals of London through collaboration with the royal family; the Victorian commitment to counter the ills of rapid industrialization, overpopulation, and poverty through charity fostered by a religious Christian fervor to "do good deeds"; and, significantly, the pronounced growth between 1861 and 1891 of charitably financed hospitals. Prochaska asserts that nursing played an indispensable role in the rise of these modern hospitals.

Prochaska also notes that by the middle of the nineteenth century, conflict

already existed between the state interventionist lobby and the view that the state's role in the health domain should be reserved for the area of public sanitation. In fact, consistently underpinning this book are the tensions between the protagonists of the voluntary system and the sympathizers of state social action.

For example, Prochaska's account of World War I and its aftermath underscores the struggles between these two forces and their effects upon the Fund. The war disrupted volunteer staffs, eroded religious faith, and generally weakened the philanthropic spirit. Escalating hospital costs, the government's impetus to centralize its economic activities, and heavy taxation of those traditionally able to make charitable donations created further economic circumstances detrimental to the Fund's work. The war reinforced for many the notion that health was a national responsibility, and Prochaska makes clear that by the 1920s, hospitals and health had become politicized as never before. During the 1930s, the Labour Party sought to centralize health services while the Liberals perpetuated Victorian traditions. This period also saw the Fund's waning relationship with the royal family, further hampering its effectiveness against threats to the voluntary hospitals.

The Fund's response to the devastating bombing of World War II was to appeal for aid and to continue its activities as best it could in the light of the loss of personnel, the closing of the Voluntary Hospital News Service, and damage to its offices. Prochaska details the emergence of the National Health Scheme (NHS) and shows how the wartime Emergency Medical Service's nationally planned and rationalized hospital service structure foreshadowed the later introduction, under the NHS, of the metropolitan hospital regions. A conflict between the forces of socialism — exhibited in the emergence of the NHS — and the Fund's commitment to the ideals of the voluntary hospital system leads Prochaska to raise doubts about the veracity of accounts claiming overwhelming public support for state intervention at the crucial time of the emergence of the British welfare state.

Among the book's few apparent shortcomings is the condensation of too much material germane to the rise of the modern hospital into one account. In certain instances, the author appears to assume the reader's prior knowledge of individuals and events; other chapters seem unnecessarily dense. Generally, more attention to the chronological framework throughout would have improved the coherence of the text.

Finally, Prochaska reveals that *Philanthropy and the Hospitals of London* was financed by the Fund, leading historian Ann Dally to raise the question of author bias. Dally questions whether there can be a fair or even valuable history if the subject of it (usually an institution) is paying for it? Other historians, in vitriolic tones, raise the same criticism. These questions seem valid enough to warrant their mention.

This book nonetheless makes a valuable contribution to the social history of the hospital in the nineteenth and twentieth centuries, with special appeal to the social historian of health in Britain and to nurse historians concerned with public health, health and hospital administration, and the role of philanthropy in the provision of care. The book would also interest any reader curious about the history of the King's Fund and philanthropy.

Particularly admirable about this work are its frequent references to nurses and the nursing profession. The incidental references to nursing invite further research highlighting the role of nursing in the relationship between the effects of the voluntary system and the role of the King's Fund in the provision of hospital patient care.

This well-researched and written account holds tenaciously to its fundamental theme, the relationship between philanthropy and the politics of socialism. The book makes clear the invaluable contribution of the King's Fund to the broad areas of health and welfare, and demonstrates, importantly, how the Fund has evolved over time to meet the demands of today's health- and welfare-focused society.

ANGELA CUSHING, PHD, RN
Senior Lecturer
School of Nursing
Queensland University of Technology
Brisbane, Queensland
Australia

Poor and Pregnant in Paris: Strategies for Survival in the Nineteenth Century
By Rachel G. Fuchs
(New Brunswick, N.J.: Rutgers University Press, 1992)

"To be poor and pregnant in Paris during the nineteenth century placed a woman in an extraordinarily difficult position." Thus begins Rachel Fuchs's social history of the experiences of a historically vulnerable population — women who were poor, uneducated, pregnant, often unmarried, and without the political or social power to influence the decisions made by others on their behalf. As a consequence, these women and their children struggled for survival in a world defined by politicians, social reformists, religious activists, and physicians. As the book's title suggests, however, unwed mothers were not without strategies for achieving some control over their reproductive lives. That these strategies — abortion, infanticide, and child abandonment — were often tragic choices, however, reflects the desperate circumstances in which the women found themselves.

Fuchs's book provides a thorough, vivid description of the life of poor women in Paris during the nineteenth century. Citing numerous statistics, Fuchs creates their world of hard work, low wages, inadequate living conditions, ignorance, and vulnerability. The cases used to emphasize the difficulty of these women's lives are not meant to garner sympathy, but rather to serve as a reminder that desperate people may make desperate decisions.

Fuchs recounts that as the numbers of poor increased in the middle of the nineteenth century, the public outrage against their immorality, especially that

of the unmarried pregnant poor, increased. Politicians joined in the condemnation of the poor's decisions to abort their unwanted pregnancies and abandon or destroy their children. Fuchs provides a thoughtful discussion of the emergence of social reforms that stemmed from the nation's outrage.

Fuchs also describes the changing nature of the country's concern, from fears of growing immorality in the population to a nationalistic concern about the vitality of the country. Faced with a shrinking population following a series of external wars and internal strife, the country's need for a viable populace partially replaced its call for a moral one. Focusing on the poor women and families, the government initiated a series of social reform policies that supported maternity care and protected children. By the end of the nineteenth century, social resources and services were available for the poor and pregnant in Paris, but to use them required negotiating a complex bureaucracy. These problems, in addition to the poor's negative view of the welfare system, served as serious barriers to true reform.

Abortions, infanticide, and child abandonment remained the poor's solution to personal and economic problems. The author provides plausible explanations for why these remedies continued to be used despite legal and social barriers.

Fuchs's text is well documented, providing a thorough list of sources for both statistics and cases. At times her use of statistics interferes with readability. However, the statistics quantify the descriptions and highlight the significance of the problem, both for the nation and the women themselves.

Fuchs suggests a parallel between the issues of the poor and pregnant of nineteenth-century Paris and the issues of the poor and pregnant in the twentieth-century United States. Certainly, today's legislators, moralists, and clergy are concerned about unwanted pregnancy, poverty, and single mothers. As our own efforts to deal with these problems have shown, in spite of providing welfare to the poor and pregnant, some desperate women still make decisions unpopular with health professionals. Thus, Fuchs's work, while not providing answers to our current questions, does provide insight into the issues that surround the questions.

Fuchs's historical examination of the specific needs and perceptions of a vulnerable population will make interesting reading for public health, social, and feminist historians. Public policy planners will particularly appreciate her analysis of which of the social, economic, and moral factors influenced the poor to participate in social reform measures. Finally, nurse educators will find the book a starting point for discussions on the role of women and the right of society to affect women's personal choices.

RITA PICKLER, PhD, RN
Assistant Professor
School of Nursing
Medical College of Virginia
Virginia Commonwealth University
Richmond, Va.

The Sanitarians: A History of American Public Health
By John Duffy
(Urbana and Chicago: Illini Books, 1992)

In *The Sanitarians: A History of American Public Health,* John Duffy more than
fulfills his purpose to outline the main developments in our public health history. Generously allowing public health to include community action to avoid
disease and other health threats as well as efforts to actively promote good
health, he has written a substantial and richly detailed account of organized and
institutional public health activity from the colonial era to the present. Indeed,
it is not inappropriate to describe *The Sanitarians* as encyclopedic: it is a comprehensive synthesis of extant scholarship in public health, to which, it should
be added, John Duffy has made major contributions, and it promises to be a
standard reference for years to come.

Although this book's range of vision is wide, the major emphasis of the
work is the "sanitary revolution" of the nineteenth century. This revolution
promoted significant advances in public health, such as improved garbage collection and street cleaning, establishment of temporary and/or permanent municipal and state boards of health, construction of new water and sewage systems, quarantine legislation, and collection of vital statistics.

Much of this salutary activity, Duffy makes clear, was stimulated by external forces, specifically the fear of epidemics of yellow fever and Asiatic cholera.
Throughout its history, Duffy reminds readers, America has had a strong reac-
tion to health crises. But equally important in the age of the reform were the
"Sanitarians," a group of dedicated reformers who spearheaded the statistical
movement, sponsored national sanitary conventions in the 1850s, and organized influential advocacy groups, such as the American Public Health Association. The sanitary conventions, Duffy argues, shifted the emphasis in public
health from quarantine to environmental concerns and thus marked the true
beginning of the American sanitary revolution. The founding of the American
Public Health Association in 1872, according to Duffy, signified the profession-
alization of public health.

Prominent among the Sanitarians were elite and well-educated physicians,
which is not surprising, Duffy notes, because medicine has played a significant
role throughout public health history. Prevailing medical concepts have always
determined what measures to use. It was the medical belief that miasmas caused
disease that sustained the sanitary revolution. Physicians also helped to organize
and staff the first municipal and state boards of health. Conversely, physicians
at times stymied the advance of public health through their reluctance to report cases of contagious diseases, citing privacy concerns and individual rights.
These conflicts between these rights and the public welfare, Duffy adds, is
another important and recurrent theme in public health history.

Nurses have been important in public health, and Duffy does acknowledge
some of their contributions, but not as fully as he might (significantly, nurses

are not included among the Sanitarians). Although Duffy does mention visiting and district nurses in the late nineteenth century, as well as rural nurses, *The Sanitarians* would be considerably strengthened if there was more recognition of nursing's role in America's public health history. Surprisingly absent from the work, for example, is any reference to the Goldmark Study; also noteworthy is Duffy's failure to include nurse recruitment among the objectives of the U.S. Sanitary Commission during the Civil War or to explore the public health work of nurses during World Wars I and II.

These omissions notwithstanding, *The Sanitarians* is a major scholarly contribution to a field that, Duffy confesses, historians have neglected. One may hope that it stimulates additional scholarship in public health, and that those who write after John Duffy bring to their work the same wisdom and understanding that he does.

JUDITH M. STANLEY, PhD
Professor of History
California State University
Hayward, Calif.

The Selling of Contraception

By Nicole Grant
(Columbus: Ohio University Press, 1992)

In *The Selling of Contraception,* Nicole Grant uses grounded theory and historical research methods to examine the personal and sociopolitical factors influencing the use of the Dalkon Shield, a notorious intrauterine device (IUD) released on the market in the late 1960s. A vital social history of the forces surrounding sexuality, reproduction, and the risks women incur to curb fertility and gain autonomy, Grant's work provides insight into the ramifications of contemporary contraceptive customs.

The Dalkon Shield was designed and marketed as the contraceptive answer for all, with spontaneous sex, near-zero pregnancy rates, and minimal side effects among its promises. Marketed without extensive testing, the Shield was promoted as superior to other IUDs; it was cited to have no systemic side effects and to meet the criteria of requiring little motivation on the part of the user. As empirical evidence of risk, injury, and higher pregnancy rates associated with the Shield emerged, physicians argued among themselves about its safety and value. Meanwhile, women continued to purchase the Shields.

Deleterious effects from the Dalkon Shield crossed socioeconomic, ethnic, and political groups. The Shield's inventor, Dr. Hugh J. Davis, denied his role in making the Dalkon Shield, withheld evidence of its side effects, concealed his financial interests for promoting the device, and perjured himself under oath for

both professional and profitable gain. The A. H. Robbins Company also with-held vital information about its efficacy and safety from the public.

Most of the women in Grant's study were unaware of debates about the Dalkon Shield and believed they were making responsible, informed choices. Women from low socioeconomic groups, with few choices, also became experi-mental recipients of the product. All of the women Grant interviewed, however, indicated a desire to protect and control personal procreative power.

Grant offers two chief reasons for the popularity of IUDs. By the late 1960s, both users and physician prescribers began to question the safety of oral contraceptives, and the drugs' unpleasant side effects prompted many to look for alternative methods that paralleled the freedom associated with oral con-traceptives. In the social arena, population control groups also advocated a global need for effective contraception requiring little motivation or control by the user. IUDs met these criteria and surfaced as the greatest hope for develop-ing countries. Grant's analysis reveals that the Dalkon Shield was valuable to the population control industry because it was cheap, difficult to expel, and easily peddled as a device that women who had never experienced a pregnancy could use effectively. Consequently, population control programs became multimil-lion dollar enterprises backed by the federal government, private foundations, and industry.

Grant's study reveals that women have paid the highest costs for the com-mercialization of reproductive control. Only successful litigation could accom-plish what years of reports of injuries and deaths failed to make happen: the removal of the Dalkon Shield from the market. Grant's analysis cautions against complacency and demands a reexamination of the attitudes shaping our re-productive and sexual lives. Grant's story of the Dalkon Shield illuminates the price paid for relinquishing reproductive control. The purchase of technology and professional knowledge hinges upon trust—trust that the technology is safe and trust that the professional community has appraised the risks and has adequately informed consumers.

Women must rethink contraceptive choice. Third-generation IUDs are on the market, and Grant reminds the reader that the risks associated with the Dal-kon Shield have been associated with most IUDs, though on a lesser scale. The injectable and implantable hormonal contraceptives now available to women also involve risks, and the devastating consequences of sexually transmitted diseases, particularly AIDS, are challenging the view that the sexual act and reproductive consequences can be separated.

For contemporary women, contraceptive practice is a dance of negotia-tion. Our partners with reproductive control include male lovers, physicians, politicians, state agencies, and the technological and corporate markets. Wom-en's desire to control fertility has been marked by risk exchange, the benefit of control against the risk of injury. The journey toward reproductive autonomy will be taken by each generation of women. *The Selling of Contraception* empha-sizes that the health of individual women must be considered as important as the overall social good and that each generation of social analysts, policy mak-ers, and contraceptive users must consciously weigh the benefits and risks for reproductive choice as a fundamental right of women.

This book will be of particular interest to historians of women, pharmaceutics, medicine, and nursing. It reveals the complex entwining of economics and professional accountability in the medical care of individuals and in society.

SALLY J. REEL, PhD, RN, FNP
Assistant Professor
School of Nursing
University of Virginia
Charlottesville, Va.

The Social Ideas of American Physicians (1776–1976): Studies in the Humanitarian Tradition in Medicine

By Eugene Perry Link
(Selinsgrove, Pa.: Susquehanna University Press, 1992)

Rudolf Virchow wrote that because illness has its origins in the social realm, medicine must also be predominately a social science. Eugene Link agrees. In this book, he advances the premise that social movements and the contexts in which noted physicians studied, lived, and practiced dramatically affected their professional lives. Though traditional biographical sources often portray physicians as isolated from the social agendas of their day, many physicians were in fact strong social activists. In this work, Link chronicles selected physicians' activist tendencies and social contributions from 1776 to 1976, and relates their actions to their particular social and political perspectives.

Link, a historical scholar, has written a cogent, well-referenced exploration of the concept that the way human beings are socialized determines their behavior, health, and destiny. Specifically, the study examines how the practice of medicine by individual doctors was strongly influenced by social and cultural contexts—not simply by the accumulation of scientific fact, as is often assumed. Link points out that prior to the Civil War, doctors were often among the most socially sensitive persons in their communities. Link describes physicians who were avid abolitionists and others whose practices were profoundly affected by context and culture. Throughout the book, Link attempts, with concrete historical data, to persuade the reader that the practice of medicine was not immune to social shaping. It is Link's view that medicine cannot be seen solely as a fact-driven, objective practice, and that physicians' professional efforts and discoveries were often colored by their social and political ideas.

In contrast to the pre–Civil War doctor, the twentieth-century physician is thought of as aloof and apolitical. In fact, the notably absent data on this group enticed Link to do his research, and he states in the preface that one of the intentions of the study was to explain the shift away from social conscience in contemporary practice. While this trend toward antihumanist practice is a fascinating phenomenon that deserves even more attention than it receives in the

book, Link speculates that one answer may be found in a reduction in quantity and quality of the interaction between professional and patient and in the trend toward specialization devoid of social understanding.

The author's main objective, of course, is not to answer this secondary question but to describe the social views and activities of medical women and men, a neglected dimension in the historical literature and a task Link fulfills richly. In doing so he makes an important contribution to the history of medicine, relying heavily on George Herbert Mead's concept of dynamic interactionism — particularly the notion of the self as arising from social experience — to support his thesis.

Link categorized each physician under consideration as one of five types: iatrocentrics, sanitationists, public health advocates, social activists who did not relate their social concerns to medical practice, or social activists who considered social concerns and medical practice intimately entwined and who acted accordingly. Two interrelated concepts — social movement and physician response — frame his ideas. Although Link sometimes fails to make fully clear how individual physicians fit into the five categories, most of the time the categorization is useful. For example, Link describes iatrocentrics as those who hold a narrow view of the world and their place in it. Link suggests that they have limited concerns and find it impossible to put themselves in the place of other people. To illustrate, Link describes Nathaniel Chapman, a physician from the late 1700s. He was the son of a Virginia Tory, and his medical practice was colored by his family's political ideas. He rejected all Jeffersonian and egalitarian ideals, and during a time of great democratic activity was opposed to the Declaration of Independence, the French Revolution, popular suffrage, and frequent elections. He led a privileged, insulated existence providing care to the elite of Philadelphia. His practice mirrored his politics, and it seemingly never occurred to Chapman that being a physician carried other duties besides those to oneself. Identification of Chapman as an iatrocentric helps the reader interpret the effect of social experience on his preferred practice pattern.

In chapters whose themes include democracy and nationalism, slavery and abolition, industrialism, gender roles, Black doctors' rights, and the public health movement, Link uses primary and secondary historical sources to flesh out social data. The book offers broad appeal for medical historical scholars, but at times can be a difficult read, packed as it is with an almost distracting abundance of information. Link's work should be of most use to social historians of medicine and to those who have more than a passing interest in psycho-history. Readers will find *The Social Ideas of American Physicians* an interesting, useful resource.

LYNN NOLAND, PhD, RN
Assistant Professor
School of Nursing
University of Virginia
Charlottesville, Va.

Red Vienna and the Golden Age of Psychology, 1918–1938

By Sheldon Gardner and Gwendolyn Stevens
(New York: Praeger Publishers, 1992)

In this text, Gardner and Stevens offer new insights into the development of psychology in Europe between the two world wars. During this period of social, religious, cultural, political, and economical unrest, Vienna emerged as the mecca of psychology. Idealistic and optimistic, psychology in this Austrian city experienced two decades of creativity and enthusiasm and sought to create a new world order.

In describing the birth of psychology during this "red" era, the authors' main goal is to emphasize that Vienna was more than just Sigmund Freud and Freudian analysis. Gardner and Stevens accomplish this by giving personable and intriguing biographies of philosophers, physicists, religious figures, and physiologists who influenced this "golden" era of psychology. The strategy of these authors is to reacquaint the reader with and to provide a different perspective of such individuals as Adolf Hitler, Theodore Herzl, and Karl Popper.

Most historical accounts of the development of psychology ignore the influence of culture on its evolution. It is impressive that Gardner and Stevens address several ethnic and cultural issues that affected the development of psychology during this era. The authors assert that although Jews were highly represented in Vienna's psychologist population, anti-Semitism permeated the thinking of some Viennese leaders.

Women also suffered from discrimination at this time. The authors discuss how Vienna's psychology theories were influenced by current attitudes that viewed females as a "sub-species" and "separate species." Most of these theories granted the "sub-species" viewpoint a biological rather than a cultural or social basis.

The authors give a considerable but appropriate amount of attention to child psychologists who believed that through educational reform and child welfare a new world order could be created. One example of this optimistic reform is the Montessori Method, which grew out of the postwar misery of Vienna's poor factory workers and their need to establish a school for their children.

In telling their story of the "Golden Age of Psychology," the authors integrate all aspects of Viennese society (e.g., politics, economics, culture, ethnicity, religion, school systems, science), thereby appealing to an audience with a wide range of disciplines and interests. Although the book is somewhat intellectual in presentation style, which may make it difficult for the lay reader to follow, the authors attempt to enhance the book's readability by presenting intriguing and surprising biographies of well-known scientists, psychologists, and philosophers. To further enhance the book's readability, the authors include a glossary to assist the reader in understanding some of the more difficult terms.

This book will interest historians of medical and nursing history, especially

those focusing on the development of psychiatry. For both the nurse researcher and clinician, it will broaden the appreciation for and understanding of trans-cultural nursing.

JOSEPHA CAMPINHA-BACOTE, PhD, RN, CS, CTN
Coordinator of Nursing Research
Upper Valley Medical Centers
Piqua, Ohio
Transcultural Consultant (Private Practice)
Wyoming, Ohio

Yellow Fever and the South

By Margaret Humphreys
(New Brunswick, N.J.: Rutgers University Press, 1992)

In *Yellow Fever and the South,* Margaret Humphreys explores the development of public health in the South as a response to recurrent epidemics of yellow fever during the nineteenth century. Occurring most frequently in the hot and humid climate of the Gulf coast, yellow fever dramatically disrupted the commerce and social activity of the region. Humphreys writes that between 1840 and 1905, yellow fever was such a burden on southern commerce that it stopped trains and bottled up ports, preventing the movement of basic merchandise from the cities to the countryside.

The introduction offers a concise summary of how the southern health movement arose from the inability of the medical community to understand or control the disease and from public outrage over the epidemic's continual threats to business, commerce, and life-style. Humphreys traces the history of the disease from 1840 until 1905, when Walter Reed and James Carroll finally convinced southern medical leaders that the mosquito was the guilty vector for transmission of the devastating disease.

Humphreys notes that until the 1880s, the South relied heavily on local and state agencies for sanitary reform and quarantine measures, resenting interference from the federal government. However, the recurrence of devastating epidemics proved these regional efforts to be inadequate. The yellow fever epidemic of 1878, for example, so severely disrupted the commercial and cultural markets of the region that the federal government at last became involved in efforts to control the importation and spread of the disease.

One of the first acts of the federal government was to initiate the National Board of Health in 1879. Dominated by northern activists, it was immediately engulfed in conflict with the U.S. Marine Service and the Louisiana State Board of Health. This strife and a lack of epidemic outbreaks in the years immediately following the national board's founding led to the loss of its funding in 1883 and its subsequent rapid disintegration.

Humphreys's major historical contribution is her explanation of what happened in the sphere of public health after the demise of the National Board of Health. After the Civil War and Reconstruction, the financial position of most southern states forced an alliance with federal agencies. At the turn of the century, southern legislators played a key role in encouraging the federal government to assume responsibility for quarantine measures and for enlarging the mandate of the old Marine Hospital to create the U.S. Public Health Service. Thus, the struggle to control yellow fever served as a major impetus for the development of federal responsibility in public health.

Humphreys uses an admirable number of primary sources to support her thesis that the South was unique in its development of public health services. However, while the book's title leads the reader to expect a comprehensive examination of the yellow fever problem in the South, the study revolves primarily around the Mississippi River valley. Humphreys allows New Orleans and Memphis to serve as microcosmic exemplars of general theories about the impact of yellow fever throughout the entire South.

Humphreys's account of yellow fever and the development of the public health movement in the South encourages us to rethink the history of public health in new terms, but the author's convoluted narrative style occasionally impedes readability. Because the narrative demonstrates neither a consistently chronological nor a thematic analysis of events, the identities of key individuals and theories and their relationships to the public health movement in the South are at times unclear.

My personal disappointment with this book was the absence of any recognition of Clara Mass's contribution to the discovery of the mosquito vector that causes yellow fever. Although great detail is given to the various etiological theories and sanitation reforms, discussion of women's roles during the epidemics is conspicuously lacking. Women are not even indexed, let alone mentioned, in the text of *Yellow Fever and the South*.

In conclusion, although Humphreys tends to use a traditional historical paradigm approach (the "great deeds of great men"), social and public health historians will gain a new perspective from the book.

QUINCEALEA BRUNK, PhD, RN
Assistant Professor
College of Nursing
Pennsylvania State University
University Park, Pa.

INDEX

GUIDELINES FOR CONTRIBUTORS

To facilitate publication of your contribution, we ask that you follow these guidelines in preparing your manuscript. For solicited articles, length guidelines and submission deadlines will be specified in the solicitation letter. Unsolicited submissions are welcome at any time and will be acknowledged promptly; manuscript length should be appropriate to the topic of the submission.

The entire manuscript (including notes, quoted or set-off text, and references) must be typed fully double spaced. Single-spaced typescripts will be returned to the author for retyping. All typescripts must be prepared with a typewriter or letter-quality computer printer. Draft-quality dot-matrix printouts will not be accepted for publication. Margins of at least one inch on all sides must be maintained. Please submit the original (ribbon) copy of the typescript and three photocopies. All pages, including reference pages, should be numbered consecutively. Please omit any author identification lines on manuscript pages to facilitate blind review.

The cover page for your article must include the following: article title (no more than two parts: title and subtitle); full names of author(s) as meant to appear in print; the address, telephone number, and fax number for the corresponding author; brief acknowledgments of support or assistance; and at least six key words or phrases to be used in subject indexing.

Up to three levels of text headings may be used in your typescript; these must be differentiated clearly in your manuscript by distinct and consistent indentations and capitalization. For questions of note style, please follow the guidelines for numbered endnotes in *The Chicago Manual of Style* (14th edition). All notes must be double-spaced and typed separately from the text (i.e., placed at the end of the article rather than as footnotes). Reference lists should be used solely to provide bibliographic data for sources cited in the text.

Tables must be typed double-spaced, each on a separate sheet, and must be accompanied by a title and/or legend. Figures (line drawings, photographs, etc.) must be submitted as black-and-white camera-ready glossy prints. All drawings, graphs, and charts must be professional-quality. Illustrations prepared with computerized graphic programs will not be accepted unless they are indistinguishable from professional-quality artwork drawn by a graphic artist. Glossy prints must be labeled on the back with the name of the article, author(s), and figure number. Photographs must be accompanied by an appropriate credit line (name of photographer, archive, or collection). Captions or legends for all figures must be typed double-spaced and provided on a sheet separate from the figures themselves. Be sure to make explicit reference to each figure and table within the text, but attach all tables and figures to the end of the typescript.

If more than 500 words of text are quoted from a scholarly book or 250 words from a scholarly article, or if a table or figure has been previously published, the article manuscript must be accompanied by written permission from the copyright owner (who is not necessarily the author of the quote, table, or figure). It is the responsibility of the author to determine who owns the copyright and to submit the appropriate permission letters. Final acceptance of the manuscript will be withheld until all necessary permission letters are received.

All correspondence concerning your submission should be sent to: Joan E. Lynaugh, Editor, *Nursing History Review,* University of Pennsylvania, 420 Guardian Drive, Room 307, Philadelphia, Pa. 19104–6096. Phone: (215) 898-4502; Fax: (215) 573-2168.

STUDIES IN HEALTH, ILLNESS, & CAREGIVING

Sick and Tired of Being Sick and Tired
Black Women's Health Activism in America, 1890-1950
Susan L. Smith

The first full-scale examination of the public health initiatives created by African Americans, the book argues that health reform was a cornerstone of early black civil rights activity in the United States. In an era of legalized segregation, health improvement was tied to the struggle for social change.
1995. 288 pp, 10 illus. Cloth, 3237-2, $34.95; paper, 1449-8, $16.95

Caring in Crisis
An Oral History of Critical Care Nursing
Jacqueline Zalumas

Zalumas examines the critical care unit during the period from the 1950s to the present. Basing her study on twenty-five interviews, she investigates the evolution of early critical care units, the intimacy of the nurse-patient interaction, and the ethical dimensions of critical care practice.
1994. 240 pp. Cloth, 3255-0, $36.95; paper, 1510-9, $14.95

Suggestions for Thought by Florence Nightingale
Selections and Commentaries
Edited by Michael D. Calabria
& Janet A. Macrae

In her unpublished work, *Suggestions for Thought*, Nightingale presented radical spiritual views, motivated by the desire to give those who had turned away from conventional religion an alternative to atheism. In this book, the editors provide the essence of Nightingale's philosophy by selecting her best-written treatments.
"Indeed, it teaches us that what we need are more real Florence Nightingales. If this book gets the attention it deserves, perhaps we will get them"—*Boston Sunday Globe*.
1994. 224 pp. Cloth, 3174-0, $34.95; paper, 1501-X, $16.95

Healing Traditions
Alternative Medicine and the Health Professions
Bonnie Blair O'Connor

O'Connor explores the interactions between conventional medicine and "vernacular" health systems, and probes the ways in which beliefs and values affect both patients' approaches to health care and health care professionals' approaches to patients.
1995. 287 pp, 12 illus. Cloth, 3184-8, $36.95; paper, 1398-X, $16.95

The Art of Asylum-Keeping
Thomas Story Kirkbride and the Origins of American Psychiatry
Nancy Tomes

"Exceptional....Easily the best history of a mental hospital in Europe or America....Tomes has achieved a remarkable fusion of exacting historical reconstruction and judicious generalization" —*Reviews in American History*.
1994. 424 pp, 19 illus. Paper, 1539-7, $15.95

Transcending AIDS
Nurses and HIV Patients in New York City
Peggy McGarrahan

In this book, a study of fifty registered nurses who have chosen to specialize in the care of HIV-infected patients in New York City, McGarrahan describes how the nurses meet the challenges of caring for HIV patients.
1994. 216 pp. Cloth, 3203-8, $31.95; paper, 1418-8, $14.95

With Child in Mind
Studies of the Personal Encounter with Infertility
Margarete Sandelowski

Using approaches from sociology, history, and women's studies, Sandelowski explores the personal experiences of infertile women and men in a social-cultural context.
1993. 320 pp. Cloth, 3197-X, $44.95; paper, 1415-3, $16.95

STUDIES IN HEALTH, ILLNESS, & CAREGIVING

Bring Out Your Dead
The Great Plague of Yellow Fever in Philadelphia in 1793
J. H. Powell; with an introduction by Kenneth R. Foster, Mary F. Jenkins, & Anna Coxe Toogood

"A ghoulishly fascinating history of Philadelphia's great plague. Historian Powell's conscientious grubbing among the records pays off with a cumulative effect of horror and heroism seldom found in the most artful fiction"—*Time*.
1993. 344 pp. Cloth, 3210-0, $31.95; paper, 1423-4, $14.95

Bargaining for Life
A Social History of Tuberculosis, 1876-1938
Barbara Bates

"I strongly recommend this book to those interested in either the history of American medicine or the problems we currently confront in battling tuberculosis....A readable, lively, occasionally moving, scholarly work filled with important insights"—*Journal of General Internal Medicine*.
1992. 456 pp, 42 illus. Paper, 1367-X, $20.95

Women at War
The Story of Fifty Military Nurses Who Served in Vietnam
Elizabeth Norman

Selected as one of the American Journal of Nursing's 1991 Books of the Year
"A powerful story about some of nursing's finest contributions. The profession is indebted to this author for her persistence and sensitivity in capturing this important piece of history"—*American Journal of Nursing*.
1990. 238 pp, 30 illus. Paper, 1317-3, $16.95

There's Nobody There
Community Care of Confused Older People
Anne Opie

Opie presents accounts of the everyday lives, in all their practical and emotional complexity, of family members who care for dependent people, specifically those suffering confusion caused by Alzheimer's disease or a related dementia.
1993. 232 pp. Paper, 1419-6, $19.95

Pictures of Health
A Photographic History of Health Care in Philadelphia, 1860-1945
Janet Golden & Charles E. Rosenberg

"This book, besides being valuable as a study of medicine in Philadelphia, could be used as an introduction to the scholarly history of modern medicine, and to the scholarly use of photographic evidence"—*Bulletin of the History of Medicine*.
1991. 224 pp, 170 b/w illus. Cloth, 8237-X, $49.95; paper, 1311-4, $32.95

Caring and Responsibility
The Crossroads Between Holistic Practice and Traditional Medicine
June S. Lowenberg

Winner of the 1989-90 Outstanding Book Award—Choice Magazine.
1989. 306 pp. Cloth, 8174-8, $38.95; paper, 1408-0, $18.95

Nurses' Work, The Sacred and The Profane
Zane Robinson Wolf
1988. 352 pp, 12 illus. Paper, 1266-5, $20.95

Clara Barton, Professional Angel
Elizabeth Brown Pryor
1987. 460 pp, 21 illus. Paper, 1273-8, $25.95

university of PENNSYLVANIA press

Quest for Conception
Gender, Infertility, and Egyptian Medical Traditions
Marcia C. Inhorn

Inhorn portrays the poignant struggles of poor, urban Egyptian women and their attempts to overcome infertility. She draws upon fifteen months of fieldwork in urban Egypt to present the stories of infertile Muslim women whose tumultuous medical pilgrimages have yet to produce the desired pregnancies.
1994. 472 pp, 24 illus. Cloth, 3221-6, $49.95; paper, 1528-1, $19.95

Providing Health Care Benefits in Retirement
Edited by Judith F. Mazo, Anna M. Rappaport, & Sylvester J. Schieber

This book identifies the challenges in providing retiree health care insurance in the current environment and under probable national health care reform scenarios.
Pension Research Council Publications. 1994. 272 pp, 35 illus. Cloth, 3270-4, $39.95

Tales from Inside the Iron Lung (And How I Got Out of It)
Regina Woods; foreword by David E. Rogers, M.D.

Tales from Inside the Iron Lung is Woods's extraordinary view of a life lived under burdens unimaginable to most people; it is also a story of the remarkable resilience of the human spirit.
1994. 160 pp, 13 illus. Paper, 1506-0, $13.95

Time to Go
Three Plays on Death and Dying, with Commentary on End-of-Life Issues
Edited by Anne Hunsaker Hawkins & James O. Ballard

This unusual book presents three prize-winning plays on the hard choices that patients, their families, and their physicians often face at the end of life.
1995. 136 pp. Paper, 1519-2, $14.95

Caring for Patients from Different Cultures
Case Studies from American Hospitals
Geri-Ann Galanti

"A welcome effort toward providing a resource both for the anthropologist teaching in a clinical setting and for the health care practitioner to consult directly"—*Medical Anthropology Quarterly.*
1991. 144 pp. Paper, 1344-0, $15.95

Women in Pain
Gender and Morbidity in Mexico
Kaja Finkler

Finkler explores the issue of why Mexican women are more likely to experience nonfatal diseases than their male counterparts.
1994. 224 pp. Cloth, 3243-7, $34.95; paper, 1527-3, $15.95

The Patient's Guide to Surgery
Edward L. Bradley III, M.D. and the Editors of Consumer Reports Books

Bradley dispels many of the myths, mysteries, fears, and anxieties surrounding the surgical experience, and provides straightforward information that will help patients make informed decisions about surgery.
1994. 256 pp, 22 illus. Cloth, 3280-1, $24.95

university of PENNSYLVANIA press

Cross Dressing, Sex, and Gender
Vern Bullough & Bonnie Bullough
"In this informative book, the Bulloughs introduce the multiple forms transvestitism and cross gendered behavior have taken historically and cross-culturally, as well as the wide variation in meanings these activities have had"—*Choice.*
1993. 400 pp. Cloth, 3163-5, $54.95; paper, 1431-5, $18.95

Postpartum Psychiatric Illness
A Picture Puzzle
Edited by James Alexander Hamilton & Patricia Neel Harberger
"*Postpartum Psychiatric Illness* should be required reading for students pursuing specialty degrees in fields related to family mental health and professionals and support leaders currently involved with prenatal and postpartum families"—*Postpartum Support, International News.*
1992. 384 pp, 29 illus. Cloth, 3137-6, $33.95; paper, 1385-8, $15.95

Intimate Adversaries
Cultural Conflict Between Doctors and Women Patients
Alexandra Dundas Todd
"[Todd] adds a much-needed perspective to recent research that has examined the micro-processes of patient-physician communication. ...A boldly comprehensive examination presented in a revealing, engaging, and personal narrative that stimulates curiosity and invites readers into her exploration"—*Contemporary Sociology.*
1989. 174 pp. Cloth, 8152-7, $38.95; paper, 1277-0, $20.95

Biting Off the Bracelet
A Study of Children in Hospitals
Second Edition
Ann Hill Beuf
"Beuf provides a challenge to students and professionals to consider the needs and humanization of hospitalized children in today's bureaucratic, profit-seeking and efficiency-driven institutions"—*Physical and Occupational Therapy in Pediatrics.*
1989. 164 pp. Paper, 1278-9, $17.95

Beauty is the Beast
Appearance-Impaired Children in America
Ann Hill Beuf
Beuf examines the stigmatization of children who deviate from acceptable American standards for physical appearance and analyzes both the effects of this stigmatization and the strategies used to cope with it.
1990. 120 pp, 7 illus. Cloth, 8234-5, $38.95; paper, 1310-6, $16.95

AMERICAN ASSOCIATION FOR THE HISTORY OF NURSING

You are invited to join the American Association for the History of Nursing, whose mission is to preserve, promote, and disseminate information about the history and heritage of the nursing profession.

What are the purposes of the AAHN?

• Stimulate national and international interest in the history of nursing, promote collaboration among its supporters, and encourage research in the history of nursing.

• Promote the development of centers for the preservation and use of materials of historical importance to nursing.

• Serve as a resource for information related to nursing history.

• Produce and distribute materials related to the history and heritage of the nursing profession.

What are the benefits of AAHN membership?

• Receive the official AAHN journal *Nursing History Review*, published annually in January and devoted to the history of nursing and health care:

Long neglected, the history of nursing has recently become the focus of a considerable amount of attention. Over the past decade, developments in the history of medicine, the history of women—particularly of women's work—and nursing itself have resulted in a new recognition of the importance of the subject.

As the official journal of the American Association for the History of Nursing, Nursing History Review *enables those interested in nursing and health care history to trace new and developing work in the field. The* Review *publishes significant scholarly work in all aspects of nursing history as well as reviews of recent books and updates on national and international activities in health care history.*

• Establish linkages with others who are ardent about the history of the nursing profession.

• Receive the AAHN quarterly *Bulletin*, which keeps you informed about calls for abstracts, fellowship and grant opportunities, conferences, book releases, and other news related to the history of nursing and the AAHN.

• Attend annual AAHN conferences where refereed papers and posters on a wide range of history of nursing subjects are presented, a book mart of historical reference material is conducted, and an auction consisting mainly of nursing memorabilia is held.

• Extend your professional insight through dialogues with colleagues.

• Learn how to compete for the annual prestigious Lavinia L. Dock and Teresa E. Christy awards, which recognize exemplary historical research and writing related to nursing history.

MEMBERSHIP/ORDER INFORMATION

Annual Dues (January 1996-December 1996):
(Subscription to **Nursing History Review** *included with membership) • Please enclose payment*

_____ Regular Member/Individual	$60.00
_____ Supporting Member/Individual	$75.00
_____ Agency	$75.00
_____ Retiree	$35.00
_____ Student	$35.00

Name   *Organization*

Address   *City*   *State*   *Zip*

Phone number (home)   *Phone number (work)*

Please photocopy this order form and send to:

American Association for the History of Nursing, Inc., P.O. Box 90803, Washington, DC, 20090-0803 • Phone number: 202-543-2127

Non-member prices for single volumes of Nursing History Review:

_____ Non-Member/Individual	$36.00
_____ Library Rate	$55.00

_____ MasterCard	Sub-total: _____
_____ VISA	Shipping/handling: $3.00 for
_____ Payment enclosed	first volume, $0.75 each add'l: _____
	TOTAL: _____

Card Number   *Expiration Date*

For back issues and orders outside the United States, please contact Julia Sawabini at (215)-898-1673.

Signature

Name   *Organization*

Address   *City*   *State*   *Zip*

Please photocopy this order form and send to: University of Pennsylvania Press, P.O. Box 4836, Hampden Station, Baltimore, MD, 21211 • Toll-free: (800) 445-9880